Dr. Paula's
Good Nutrition Guide

for Babies,
Toddlers, and Preschoolers

Paula M. Elbirt, M.D., FAAP

PERSEUS PUBLISHING

Cambridge, Massachusetts

Copyright © 2001 by Paula M. Elbirt, M.D.

Note: The information in this book is true and complete to the best of our knowledge. This book is intended only as an informative guide for those wishing to know more about nutrition for children. In no way is this book intended to replace, countermand, or conflict with the advice given by your child's own pediatrician. The ultimate decision concerning care should be made between you and your child's doctor. We strongly recommend you follow his or her advice. The information in this book is general and is offered with no guarantees on the part of the author or Fisher Books. The author and publisher disclaim all liability in connection with the use of this book. The names and identifying details of people associated with events described in this book have been changed. Any similarity to actual persons is coincidental.

Cataloging-in-Publication data for this book is available from the Library of Congress.
ISBN 0-55561-305-5

Perseus Publishing is a member of the Perseus Books Group.
Find us on the World Wide Web at http://www.perseuspublishing.com

Perseus Publishing books are available at special discounts for bulk purchases in the United States by corporations, institutions, and other organizations. For more information, please contact the Special Markets Department at the Perseus Books Group, 11 Cambridge Center, Cambridge, MA 02142, or call (800) 255-1514.

Text design by Cindy Young
Set in 11-point Sabon

First printing, June 2001
1 2 3 4 5 6 7 8 9 10—04 03 02 01

Dr. Paula's
Good Nutrition Guide

ALSO BY PAULA M. ELBIRT, M.D.

Dr. Paula's House Calls to Your Newborn

365 Ways to Get Your Child to Sleep
(with Linda Lee Small)

The *Seventeen* Guide to Sex and Your Body
(with Sabrina Solin)

A New Mother's Home Companion
(with Linda Lee Small)

Contents

Introduction

As I was walking between examination rooms recently, I wished that I could introduce the family in exam room A to the family in exam room B. The children in both rooms had food-related "issues"—one was a picky eater and the other was what I dub a "dessert monster." Both children had a couple of rather desperate parents. I knew that if the two families could meet, they would be greatly reassured to know they were not alone.

A good deal of my practice consists of listening to parents' questions—often those I've answered many, many times before. Particularly on weekends and evenings, parents will call apologetically ("I know this really isn't an emergency, but I wanted to run this by you"). Parents often need the answers to their questions at the time they occur. ("This may sound silly, but my four-year-old son will eat only 'white' food this week. Is that normal?") As one parent said wistfully, "Dr. Paula, I really wish all this information were in a book and then I wouldn't have to keep bothering you." I wrote this book with these parents in mind.

I want to point out that although this book is divided into sections by age, every parent must keep one overriding fact in mind: *No two children are alike*. Children are born with temperaments. Some are picky eaters from birth; others eat anything not nailed down. Generally your child will arrive in this world fitting more or less into one of the following categories:

- *The grazer.* This is a particularly common style for toddlers who "munch" as they toddle about.
- *The ruminator.* Ruminators are children who put food in their mouths, but hardly ever swallow. (It's an hour later, and the mashed potatoes are still in his mouth.) This child may become a picky eater.
- *The barracuda.* This eater rolls through the table at dinnertime—maybe eating off of every family member's plate. This child can consume large amounts of food and may be destined to be obese.
- *The stuffer.* As the name implies, the child eats quickly (as if a sibling is poised to come by and steal his food) and stuffs lots of different foods into his mouth. (Stuffers often complain of stomachaches.) This child may end up being an overeater.

It's part of the nature of children that eating habits often change as the child grows older—a two-year-old grazer may transform into a four-year-old barracuda. Not to worry!

The most critical "ingredient" in a book about nutrition is actually a sense of humor. Always bring along your sense of whimsy. To that end I offer an anonymous gift from my web site. Visit my web site at www.drpaula.com and click on "Ask the Pediatrician," then go to "Topics" and click on "Diet, Toddler" to read the Toddler Miracle Diet. Enjoy and, of course, "take with a grain of salt."

PART ONE

How to Feed Your Child

1

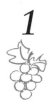

Food for Thought:
The Ten Commandments

*M*eet Jane and John Smith. (The names have been changed to protect the nutritionally challenged.) You know them; they probably live next door to you or down the block. The Smiths have four children under the age of five. I'm their pediatrician. The youngest is ten-month-old Tommy, their pride and joy. He's a "no-brainer" in terms of feeding. Jane reports that Tommy lets her know *exactly* when he is hungry. "All he has to do is cry. I feed him and he's happy." In fact, Tommy is so easy compared to the other kids that Jane smiles a lot at him and says, "Mommy loves you" with each bite of food.

Then there are the two-and-a-half-year-old twin toddlers, Jack and Jill. Jack eats everything in sight—if it's not nailed down, it's swallowed. Jane is a little concerned about how much Jack eats. She says, "Lately I have tried rewarding him when he eats food like veggies, and I take away TV time when he eats too much junk." Jack has been drinking skim milk since his first birthday. In fact, he still drinks six bottles a day!

Jack can often be found eating in front of the TV with his dad, John. At the end of the day, John often reaches for the remote and sometimes for a can of soda. He loves this opportunity to bond with Jack, and occasionally baby Tommy is right beside them on the couch as well. Jack likes to share chips with his dad, so Jane always makes sure to leave out a bowl of nachos.

Jill, the other twin, is a picky eater. Make that a *very* picky eater. Some days it seems that all she eats is "round food"—a few Cheerios and a couple of berries. Mom lets Jill have as many bottles of milk as she wants because she figures, "Calories are calories, and I know she's got to be healthy from all that milk."

The preschooler, Lilly, is what I call a perfect "four." At four years old she weighs forty pounds and is forty inches tall. Like her little sister, she has some unusual eating habits, like insisting that her sandwich be cut into perfect stars. And she is also your classic "dessert monster." Many nights the only food she will eat is dessert. Even though Lilly isn't skinny, mom is worried that she could starve. "If she eats dessert, then at least she's getting some calories. Sometimes she won't eat all day unless she gets dessert first. One day I was so scared, I actually promised her a new Barbie doll if she would just swallow some peas."

Recently mom brought in all four kids for checkups. When I asked if she had any particular concerns, Jane confessed, "I know all kids should eat three meals a day, but my kids never seem interested in food when I'm ready to serve it. I think Tommy and Jack are basically OK—they both eat a lot. The ones I'm really worried about are Jill and Lilly. Do you have any advice?"

Oh, yes I do! First, Jane and John have to take a giant step out of the kitchen to reassess what's happening. You know what they say about "good intentions." The Smiths are paving their way right down the road to nutritional disaster.

Parents need to understand that bad eating habits translate into serious health issues over time. Good nutrition takes more than just knowing the five basic food groups. (Although they do matter—that's why Chapter 10 of this book is devoted to them.) Over the years, I've collected a list of common mistakes parents make when it comes to feeding their children. I call these "Food for Thought: The Ten Commandments." See if you can guess which rules the Smiths have broken. (Hint: Think "perfect ten.")

1. Thou shall not confuse food with love.

Food is *not* love. When a baby is born, he is quickly brought to the breast to feed. We learn early that to feed is to sustain life. Feeding, in fact, is the focus of the earliest infant-parent bond. And that's a very good thing; it's "mother" nature at her best.

For some parents, "food as love" remains the singular means of demonstrating their love. This limited view can establish troublesome patterns that last a lifetime, often accompanied by statements such as, "Eat for mommy," or "I made this just for you." If the child doesn't eat, then mom may think, "You don't love me," or "I'm not loving you well enough." The actual food gets lost in the picture. Children pick up the message and may conclude, "I want to be loved, so I need to eat more."

Overeating becomes natural, and the response to the baby's signal to stop eating gets overridden. Jack and Tommy Smith have both learned how to "eat for mommy." In fact, Jack is also eating for daddy with those chips. Jane would be better off letting Tommy feed himself instead of telling him what a good boy he is while she spoons more food into him.

"Food as love" starts out as part of an essential need for survival. However, don't make food your primary expression of love after the first few months of your child's life.

2. Thou shall not use food to control behavior.

It starts out innocently. When Jane feeds Tommy, she gets a real charge out of his happiness. When he seems reluctant to eat, she "plays airplane" with the spoon, bringing the mashed potatoes in for a landing. Tommy eagerly cooperates and opens his mouth . . . even though he isn't really hungry. Then mom smiles! Incidentally, this is also how Tommy learns to control *mom's* behavior with food.

For some, this scenario, which is replayed over and over, may become the root of serious food disorders later in adolescence. Girls are particularly susceptible to this power/control combination and may use it later in the form of anorexia and bulimia.

Lilly, the Smiths' four-year-old, probably learned early how to manipulate her parents with food. She knows how very important food is to mom and dad, and now she can even bargain for a new Barbie doll just by agreeing to eat. If she hasn't eaten in a couple of days, she can up the ante. In short, Lilly controls her environment by controlling the food she eats. It surely doesn't help that Grandma lets Lilly know that she thinks she is a little heavy (see number 8).

3. Thou shall not punish or reward your child with food.

Bad behavior should not result in going to bed without supper. If Jack kicks Aunt Marge, that shouldn't mean he doesn't get dessert. (See number 6.) On the other hand, if you offer food as a reward for good behavior, you'll have a child who will eagerly look for that reward. The behavior that you wanted to reinforce gets repeated only because of the reward. If you instruct, "Say 'please' and 'thank you' and then you will get dessert," you are teaching your children to overeat, not to be polite.

We are a culture surrounded by food rewards. As you walk down the street, store after store beckons with varieties of donuts, popcorn, candy—you name it. We even take "coffee breaks." In Europe, workers stop for rest breaks. In Japan, it's a time to stretch and exercise. We use the break to stuff ourselves with food because we were taught very early to use food as reward.

4. Thou shall not turn the dining-room table into a battlefield.

Although mealtime can be a wonderful opportunity for sharing news, learning about nutrition, and satisfying the appetite, too often it is also the location of heated struggles. ("Don't talk with your mouth full." "You are not leaving this table until you eat all of your vegetables.") Your children should never dread mealtime. Good manners, though important, are best taught away from your table. Save the "lectures" for "tea parties" or outings to the diner with your preschooler. Jane may not like it when Lilly pushes food around on her plate while sitting with her elbow up to her ear, but she doesn't need to comment on it. She can model good manners without saying a word, and eventually Lilly will mirror the good manners right back.

5. Thou shall not overreact to a picky eater.

The most common eating problem among young children is so-called picky eating. At the right age, it is absolutely normal behavior, but most parents still overreact to it. It is predictable for a two-year-old to be concerned suddenly about the shape, form, and color of his food and to reject it if it isn't "just so." It's his job to learn about his world this way, and it's natural for him to throw a tantrum when it doesn't work out just as he wants.

   Jane is obviously concerned about Jill and is bemoaning the fact that she used to be such a good eater. She still *is* a "good" eater, for a toddler. Jane needs to let up on the pressure she is directing toward Jill. Otherwise Jill will stand in her big sister's sneakers and start controlling her parents with food.

6. Thou shall understand that children don't need as much food as you think they do.

Like most parents, Jane is overestimating just how much food her children need. Ironically, the children she considers to be eating well are actually overeating. Infants need more food than toddlers do. Babies actually grow to be almost three times their birth weight by the time they become toddlers. After that, growth slows down dramatically, and new skills start rolling in. Toddlers learn to run, jump, sing, dance, say "no," and burn off lots of calories. But they actually eat very little. Somehow nature allows for this system to work.

   Some toddlers who eat a lot due to parental pressure and not because of their own hunger pangs are at risk for future obesity. A good rule of thumb is to think in terms of "one teaspoon's worth" a day for every two pounds your child weighs. So a twenty-pound toddler will not need more than about ten teaspoons of food a day.

7. Thou shall not get hung up on three meals a day.

Three meals a day doesn't make sense to the inner workings of most children. It really exists only to fit our adult work schedule. Parents will say, "I don't understand; he played hard all day and then didn't even eat much for supper." Or, "He slept all day, but he woke up hungry." Indeed, there is no direct match between energy spent and the need for more food, especially during the toddler years.

I often explain to parents that children aren't automobiles and food isn't like gasoline. When you drive your car, you know you will get, let's say, twelve miles to the gallon. You put twenty gallons of gasoline in your car and can reasonably expect to go about 240 miles before needing to refuel; if you forget, your car will stop dead in its tracks. That's not the way children "run." Children grow in spurts.

I have heard parents say, "He got up this morning and I swear he grew three inches overnight." One day he may need more "fuel" and other days less. Or I'll hear, "Something is wrong with my child; he hasn't eaten in three days but he keeps on going, like a battery." I say, "Call me in six days." I rarely hear back, because during the second three days the kid eats like crazy. I also occasionally get calls that report, "Now Max is eating everything in sight." I say, "Remember when Max didn't eat for three days? This is catch-up." The spurts in appetite are related to spurts in growth. Yes, some kids need to eat a little bit all day long, but others don't need more than one meal a day. Be prepared. Your kitchen doesn't need to be open for business three times every day.

8. Thou shall not fear fat in your infant.

Jack's nutritionally misguided parents put him on skim milk at age one because of fear of fat. Giving skim milk to a hearty toddler is not only unwise but can lead to nutritional deficiencies and neurological problems. There are also some cases of "insufficient feeding syndromes" where a mother actually withholds food from her infant in an effort to keep him slim.

Many parents have bought into the notion that "you really can't be too thin." Just because you have a chubby baby doesn't mean he will be a fat adult. It is understandable that given today's obsession with controlling cholesterol, parents want to head off future health problems. This can lead a parent to conclude that a child should be fed only lean cuisine. Trust me, "baby fat" is a good thing, both literally and metaphorically.

9. Thou shall not create a dessert monster.

Dessert monsters are made, not born. Once they take up residence, they are hard to banish. Lilly is now a full-fledged dessert monster who refuses to budge until she is fed a sweet. Ten-month-old Tommy is a monster in training—he does not need the pudding Jane offered to top off his meal. Jane needs to understand that Tommy won't even notice that he didn't get dessert. Nutritionally, dessert is usually some form of junk food and concentrated sugar. But it's presented with special fanfare, often to children who are no longer even hungry.

Dessert is often offered as a reward for good behavior or for having eaten everything on the child's plate. How smart is that? ("We'll give you some junk food later because you ate healthfully now.") And never get into the habit of training your child to eat one food (vegetables) in order to earn another one (pudding).

That doesn't mean you should never give kids dessert. If your family's tradition includes somebody's great baking on special occasions, then go for it every now and then. There is no harm in an occasional special dessert, especially if the family history doesn't include obesity.

10. Thou shall not mistake calories for nutrition.

Your child needs not only calories but also a variety of foods that increase as your child gets older. Your child needs nutritional diversity in order to get all the good nutrients that nature offers. Parents may add up a day's worth of cookie calories and erroneously convince themselves that at least they provided "enough" calories, even if they weren't spread out over the various food groups.

Jane thinks that Jill is getting good nutrition because she gets seven bottles of milk a day. She is filling up a picky eater with milk, and that's not good nutrition. Jane is also breaking commandment number 9. She is encouraging another dessert monster to haunt the family. The quality of the food your child eats *does* count.

Although the Smiths have broken every commandment on my informal list, they are not so different from many of the families in my practice. Without knowing the essential rules, even loving parents make mistakes in the kitchen. Keep these ten commandments in mind as you move through the chapters ahead.

2

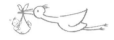

Infants:
The Beginning

Dear Dr. Paula,

I have decided that life as a baby is grand. People feed
you until you are full, everyone wants you to gain
weight, and it is socially acceptable and even
encouraged for you to belch loudly in public.
Everyone thinks that you are cute, and everyone
wants you to go to sleep. What a life!

Annie, Suzie's mom

Dear Annie,

*Infants do live blissful existences, if they are lucky
enough to have loving parents. In case envy gets the
better of you, remember that right after infancy, the
toddler years set in, and that's not an easy period for
anyone involved. Try to hold on to some of the joys
of infancy in the coming years. And right from the
beginning, don't always comfort your baby with your
breast or a bottle. Choose ways to comfort your baby
that include hugs and kisses.*

Breast Is Best

There's no escaping the truth: Breast is best for infant feeding. Breast-feeding is superior to any other method of feeding your newborn because breast milk is ideally suited for baby's growth and development. Breast milk contains the "memory" of protection against many diseases. That protection is the product of the mother's own health experiences: years of combating life's inevitable bouts with viruses and bacteria. Mom's immune system has a memory bank of antibodies that she passes along through her breast milk. (Antibodies are proteins in the blood that produce immunities against certain microorganisms.)

Breast milk has many other advantages for baby. Breast milk has a stimulating effect on baby's bowel. It's a natural stool softener, making it easier for the baby to pass the first stools, known as meconium. That's why breast-fed babies have such "lovely" soft, mushy stools, often with every feed. If the mother has reasonable nutrition, her breast milk is rich in calories and perfectly balanced in nutrients. Second only to life itself, breast milk is the best gift you can give your child.

New mothers often ask me what kind of milk is best: the first milk, the middle milk, or the hind milk? I respond that *all* the milk is good for baby. The first milk, called colostrum, is highest in antibodies and fat. It's a thick, yellow milk, although sometimes it looks almost transparent. You might call colostrum the "crème de la crème" of breast milk. It's unmatched in

FYI: Breast-fed babies eat every two to three hours and formula-fed babies are fed every three to four hours. Breast milk is always available and it's free.

function and importance. Then follows the "ordinary" milk, which looks like bluish milk.

Although it can't be seen with the eye, the milk that baby sucks in the first few minutes is different from the milk that comes after a child has been sucking for a good fifteen to twenty minutes. The first milk is highest in immunologic properties and carbohydrates, and the hind milk is highest in fat and protein. For this reason, once breast-feeding is established, babies should be allowed to suck for as long as practical to reap the many benefits breast milk offers.

I encourage mothers to continue breast-feeding right into the period when solid foods will be introduced, at about five to six months of age.

How long to breast-feed

It is best to breast-feed throughout the entire first year of the infant's life, but the most critical period is the first three months. The baby's own immune system begins to kick in and learns to make its own antibodies at about the age of two months. At the same time, the amount of antibodies and immune factors that are transmitted through breast milk begins to decline. I encourage mothers to continue breast-feeding right into the period when solid foods will be introduced, at about five to six months of age.

What mommy eats affects breast milk quality

Since breast milk is a product of the mother, it is influenced by what the mother is eating. That includes medication and alcohol as well as foods. That can present a problem, especially if a

FYI: Breast-feeding and Herbs

Although many herbs have been advertised to stimulate milk production, few have been proven to do so by scientific study. Moreover, some of these "galactagogues," such as fenugreek, have side effects that range from diarrhea to dangerously lowered blood-sugar levels. Breast-feeding moms should be cautious in their choice of herbal teas as well. For example, comfrey may be dangerous and lead to liver failure in baby, and its use is outlawed in several countries. Another herb, sage, is known to depress milk production. Read labels very carefully.

woman has delayed a medical treatment or procedure during pregnancy and also wants to breast-feed. In addition, if a breast-feeding mother smokes, the infant is "puffing" away and getting nicotine as well.

Allergies and breast milk

If you are breast-feeding, you can eat just about anything that's good for you. If your baby seems a little uncomfortable when she feeds, cut back on your own consumption of cow's milk and other dairy products. *Babies are meant to drink the protein found in human breast milk, and calves are meant*

The baby may have an allergic reaction to something mom eats, but an allergy to human breast milk is virtually unheard of.

Some "Safe" Herbs for Breast-Feeders

These may stimulate production of breast milk:

- Evening primrose
- Mint
- Rose hips (lots of vitamin C)
- Orange spice
- Ginger
- Lemongrass
- Borage (pain reliever)
- Thistle (caution: some reports of nausea)

Other safe breast-feeding stimulants, not scientifically proven:

- Hops
- Oatmeal
- Marshmallow seed

to drink the protein of cow's milk. To avoid having cow protein in *your* breast milk, don't have a lot of cow dairy in *your* diet. Contrary to common belief, you don't need to drink milk to make milk. Remember that cows eat grass, and they make plenty of milk!

What about nutritional supplements?

Even if you are breast-feeding, your newborn may need certain nutritional supplements, depending on your health and lifestyle.

Breast-fed babies may need supplementation with vitamins A and D because breast milk can be deficient in those vitamins. Vitamin D, in particular, requires mom to have a lot of exposure to sunlight, but because of the warnings regarding sun exposure, some mothers may be vitamin-D deficient and their milk will be as well. (Sunlight is needed to process and use vitamin D, and vitamin D is needed to use calcium to build strong bones.)

Formula

If a baby is not being breast-fed, the most common alternative is to use a commercially made formula. It *is* possible to make formula on your own, but today you would be ill advised to bother because commercially available formulas are varied enough and nutritionally standardized to work very well for

Special Ingredients

Two particular fatty acids that are present in mother's milk—aracadonic acid and DHA—are now present in formula in several European countries. These fatty acids have a positive impact on the child's neurological development. In recent research, children on the formula with those two fatty acids added did better on development tests and at eighteen months had better memory and social skill assessments. As yet, the FDA has not given approval, but look for these fatty acids to be added to U.S. formulas in the near future.

FYI: When you use formula, count on giving baby twenty calories for every ounce he consumes. Calories within breast milk vary slightly, depending on which portion of the milk the baby is drinking and the mother's own nutrition.

most babies. Formula is not just a container of regular milk with some sugar and oil in it. On the contrary, formula today duplicates mother's milk to the greatest possible extent.

Formula is made with everything your baby needs, including iron, and has many essential vitamins added to it as well. For the most part, there is little reason why a formula-fed baby would be given vitamins (though they often are). Soon we may even be using molecularly engineered formula with protective antibodies already added.

Formula stages

Formula manufacturers are constantly reformulating and improving formulas as they increase their understanding of the composition and changes in breast milk that occur over time. That's why formula products are now being offered in stages. There are subtle differences in each stage intended to adapt to infants' nutritional needs the way breast milk does. It's not entirely clear whether the adaptations are enough to merit the extra cost of these formulas. With time and research, formulas may become so well tailored to infant nutritional needs as to compare very well to breast feeding. In the amounts and kinds of fat, protein, minerals, and vitamins, manufacturers are getting better and better at "matching" breast milk in the laboratory.

~

Preemies

Premature babies are often sent home on formula that is higher in calories and made especially to help replace deficits common to prematurity. This period requires close cooperation with the baby's pediatrician and a nutritional specialist in newborn feeding issues. If the new mother is breast-feeding, human milk fortifiers can be used to help tiny babies gain weight. Premature babies also need supplementation of specific nutrients and minerals. Although I usually advise parents that kids don't need to take vitamins and minerals, premature babies do. They need extra iron, zinc, magnesium, and a variety of vitamins because they missed out on a lot of intrauterine development.

Three categories of formula

- Formulas based on cow's milk are the most common type of formulas. These formulas replicate breast milk using cow's milk as the base. The advantage of cow-milk formula is that it contains the amino-acid chains that are found in all mammal milk products, including human breast milk.
- The second category is based on soybean protein (we call it soy formula). It differs in many ways from the composition of formula based on cow's milk. A variety of important fats and sugars are added to make it adequate for feeding infants. For children who are not

Formula Brand Names

Cow-milk formula: Enfamil, Similac
Soy-based formula: ProSobee, Isomil, Nursoy, Soy-a-lac
Hydrolyzed protein formula: Nutramigen and Alimentum
Lactose-free cow-milk formula: LactoFree, EnfamilDF

breast-fed and who cannot tolerate cow-milk formula, soy-based formula is currently the recommended substitute.

- The third category is hydrolyzed protein formula for babies who have difficulties digesting soy and cow-milk formulas. These are also referred to as hypoallergenic formulas. A family with a strong history of allergies might benefit from starting their baby on a hypoallergenic formula. These formulas are partially metabolized and, in some cases, are lactose-free, making digestion easier.

FYI: If you *and* your baby's daddy are both allergic to cow-milk protein, there's a very good chance your child will be allergic as well. At least 15 percent of people who are allergic to cow-milk protein are also allergic to soy protein. In this situation, your pediatrician will probably recommend the third category—formula that is partially hydrolyzed.

When should I change formulas?

- *Baby could be allergic to cow's milk.* If your baby cries with feedings and produces occasional blood-tinged stool, he is likely to be suffering from milk protein allergy. Other signs include vomiting and a blotchy hive-like rash. If you see these signs, consult your pediatrician about it immediately. If your baby has discomfort every time he eats—he cries, pulls up his legs, turns red in the face, and throws up—call your baby's doctor. This may be due to the formula that your baby is drinking, but it could also relate to medical conditions such as reflux or lactose intolerance. Your doctor can help make the diagnosis.

- *Baby could be lactose intolerant.* Many babies are gassy, but gassy *and* uncomfortable may mean that your baby is lactose intolerant. Although it is often suspected, it is not very common. Lactose-free cow-milk formulas are available, although they are not as easy to find and tend to cost more. Soy formula does not contain lactose. Unfortunately soy tends to constipate babies, so a parent will lament: "I traded a gassy baby for a constipated baby."

  You might switch to that third category—hydrolyzed formulas. These are made by breaking down the protein component so that the child who is allergic to the protein in cow's milk will be able to digest it more easily. It still originates from cow's milk and is more similar than soy-based formula to human milk, which is the "gold standard." It is also harder to find and more expensive, but certainly worth trying if it relieves suffering. The not-so-good news is that infants who use this formula smell "funny." You can always tell a Nutramigen or an Alimentum baby by his distinctive odor. Also, be prepared for stools that will be very watery and dark green. This is expected and does not mean anything is wrong or that baby is not getting enough nutrients.

- *Babies have taste buds, too!* Why else might you change formulas? Well, let's say your baby is not interested and just won't drink it. Its flavor may not appeal to her. We don't know everything about infants' taste buds, but we do know they work, because babies grimace and spit out foods with certain tastes. If your baby repeatedly spits out the same brand of formula, maybe she just doesn't like it. Try a different brand, or try changing from cow-milk to soy-based formula.

How do I know baby has enough to drink?

Make sure your baby eats enough to produce at least six wet diapers and about one poop a day. That translates into about six to ten feedings a day in the first six months of life.

As your baby gets bigger, you may think that she needs to drink ever-increasing amounts of formula, but that's not the case. A newborn will drink approximately 16 to 24 ounces a day in the first week or two, and then the amount gradually increases. By the time they are two months old, most infants take an average of 32 ounces of formula a day—some more, some less. However, parents who think, "My baby is getting bigger, so she must need more calories" can be misled into overfeeding their baby. Your newborn should gain one to two pounds per month, doubling her weight by about six months.

~

Don't add cereal to baby's bottle!

Some parents add cereal to the bottle at a very early age, hoping to get their baby to sleep through the night. This is not a good idea. This often causes indigestion and then the baby is definitely "up." Adding food too soon is also an invitation to allergies, asthma, eczema, and other undesirable outcomes like obesity. *Never add cereal to the bottle, and don't add solids to your baby's diet until your infant is almost six months old.*

Tips for feeding baby by bottle

Babies should suck in the semi-upright position and avoid excessive pacifier use. This is believed to help prevent ear infections. In addition, bottles should never be "propped," that is, left unattended in your baby's mouth. Your infant could choke on the pooled milk, and it is also an invitation for tooth decay.

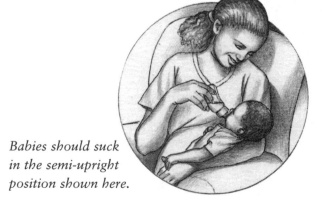

Babies should suck in the semi-upright position shown here.

Bonding and Feeding

From the start, it's important that when you feed your baby, whether by breast or by bottle, you make feeding a very positive experience. Specifically, when feeding your newborn, hold her so your two faces are only about twelve inches apart and you can focus exclusively on each other. That happens to be exactly the distance your newborn can see best. This position nurtures your developing bond with your baby. Your baby learns that love is a part of the feeding with your every smile or warm gaze and gesture. The two of you form a safety cocoon: your baby in your arms, your eyes locked on each other. (This is definitely one of those "Kodak" moments!)

As your infant approaches three, four, and five months, you will no longer need to stay completely focused on each other while feeding. In fact, it is a good idea to allow other "things" to happen—simple things like music in the background, singing, or reading aloud to match your baby's developmental stage. As baby matures, some feeding should just be "business"—brief and to the point. As baby gets older, she will get more interested in the outside world, start unfolding like a newly emerging butterfly, and begin looking around beyond the nipple. That is how it should be.

I have seen parents cover their baby's head while feeding to eliminate outside stimulation. That may be a good thing for the first few weeks, warm and cuddly. But by the third month, that habit would make it hard for baby to look outward and observe the bigger world. By baby's third month, it's time to remove the cocoon so that you don't teach baby that feeding and being fed is her entire world.

Dear Dr. Paula,

My two-month-old daughter Kayla is driving us crazy! She spit up when we gave her the formula we brought home from the hospital, so we switched to a soy kind. She still spits up, only now she's also constipated. I've tried switching back to the first brand—the kind without iron in it—but it made no difference. *Help!* Oh, and she also drinks tons and is gaining weight really well.

Kayla's mom

Dear Kayla's mom,

You are in good company. Most babies spit up, and soy formula is known to cause hard stools. It's possible your little one is really fine and just needs you to be more patient. Unless she is in pain, I would stop switching formula and keep her on one with iron. Despite rumors you might have heard, iron in the formula does not constipate your baby. Whatever you do, cherish your little one.

3

Introducing Solid Foods

Dear Dr. Paula,

Today Audrey sat in the high chair for the first time
and ate an entire jar of sweet potatoes. She opened
her mouth and gulped it down, and she cried when
the jar was finished. It is the first time she has had
anything other than rice cereal and formula!

Audrey's mom

Dear Audrey's mom,

*Your six-month-old is making all the right "moves."
Keep in mind how clearly she is communicating her
hunger at this age, and be sure to respond to her
messages—in this case, by opening up another jar of
food. And don't forget to wear a raincoat at feeding
time! Things are going to get very messy now.*

Until now, feeding your infant has been relatively uncomplicated.
Everything your baby needed was available from breast milk or
a can of formula. Even the quantities she took in had become
predictable. Along with your baby's increasing levels of

development, her nutritional requirements are about to mature. Chances are you have been eyeing the great variety of baby food jars at your grocery store for months. Now is the time to go shopping.

When to Start Solids

It isn't always so easy to decide exactly when *your* baby is ready for something more than milk. Even the experts are a bit vague on this issue. The timing depends on your particular baby's level of physical and developmental maturation. Some babies are ready for solids at four months; most are not ready until closer to six months of age.

Physically speaking, your baby should have at least doubled his birth weight or weigh more than fifteen pounds before starting solid foods. Before this time, your baby's digestion isn't prepared to handle any nutrition other than milk. Almost anything else is bound to end up causing trouble, even if your baby looks as though she is enjoying herself. Some of these troubles can result in lifelong allergies or become the basis for obesity later on. At the very least, you are likely to have a very unhappy infant with a stomachache or an infant who develops an aversion to new tastes, which

Physically speaking, your baby should have at least doubled his birth weight or weigh more than fifteen pounds before starting solid foods.

can set you back for weeks if you start too soon. (The only one who may approve is grandma, who has decided you are otherwise starving your baby.) Another common reason that parents start solids too soon is the mistaken belief that feeding solids will help the child sleep through the night. Nothing could be further from the truth!

Another physical sign that your baby is ready for solids is teething. This heralds the approaching appearance of the first teeth. When your baby gnaws eagerly on a teether, she is learning the physical process necessary for chewing on solid foods. The development of baby's mouth and tongue muscles that results from the teething process is in sync with changes that are also occurring in baby's digestive system now. Even baby's intestines are getting ready for the new foods.

At the same time, baby's muscles and bones are also preparing for the big moment. Your baby needs to be able to sit up and control her upper body in order to help the internal processes of digestion.

All systems being ready to go, you can imagine this new little person sitting up, mouth open, hands ready to grab at this new experience of eating. Even your baby's emotional state comes into play. Your six-month-old is aware of her surroundings, and she is communicating with sound and facial expressions in increasingly sophisticated ways. Everything about this baby says, "What's for dinner?"

How to Feed, What to Feed

The first time you feed your baby solids may be worth recording. After all, this is the beginning of a new level of relationship between your baby and the world. These first spoonfuls are the beginning of a long nutritional journey.

I tell my moms to load up the camera, wear a raincoat, and carry an umbrella. Inevitably, baby's first culinary attempts will be sloppy. Most of the first efforts will land on a bib or the floor or even the family pet. Your baby has to learn, by practice, how to keep new textures in the mouth and move them down her throat. This "skill" is very

I tell my moms to load up the camera, wear a raincoat, and carry an umbrella.

different from the sucking she did so well in the first six months. It's important for you not to assume that your baby doesn't like a particular food just because more seems to come out than goes down. Gradually, over time, you will learn your baby's signals so that you will know which are her favorite foods and which she would rather do without.

High chairs and spoons

Always feed your baby in a high chair that is secure and stable. In the beginning, baby has a lot to concentrate on: staying upright, keeping her hands out of the way of incoming food, and getting her mouth to open and close in rhythm. Use any small spoon to feed her that fits comfortably in her mouth. It's helpful to have an extra spoon or two available to occupy baby's own curious hands.

Keep distractions to a minimum

The job will be easier if there are quiet surroundings and few distractions for parent and child. Once she gets the hang of it, it may be fun for her to eat with her older siblings, but for starters, make it dinner for one. Don't get into the bad habit of leaving the television on in the background. Not only are the food messages unhealthy, but eating while distracted is an invitation to overeating.

Warning: Do not put solids into your baby's bottle! This practice may come from the wish to make feeding less messy or from a time when solids were introduced too early and baby wasn't ready for a spoon. Not only is this developmentally inappropriate, but it can also be dangerous to your baby's health. Solids in a closed, warm bottle of milk are likely to become a germ magnet quickly.

Try one new food at a time

Often parents ask, "Does it really matter what I feed her? Can't I just offer anything as long as I grind it up?" For most children, this results in gastric distress, at the very least. For some, it could cause severe discomfort and even trigger allergic reactions, so proceed slowly and carefully to introduce foods to your baby. The usual rule is to feed your child one new food at a time for at least two to three days, twice a day, while looking out for a reaction.

The usual rule is to feed your child one new food at a time for at least two to three days, twice a day, while looking out for a reaction.

Two teaspoons, twice a day, for two days

Let your child have only a couple of teaspoons of food each time you feed her. After you have figured out that the food is not causing distress or allergy, start thinking in terms of letting your baby make the decision of how much food she wants to eat. When she turns her face away from the spoon, give her a minute. She may not be done swallowing the last mouthful.

Then offer food again when she turns her face back to you with her mouth open. A second turndown probably means it's time to put the food away.

When baby stops eating, do *not* interpret this as a cue to start the "airplane game." Be aware of the cues your baby is sending and be respectful, not overbearing.

First Foods

Cereal

The easiest thing for children to digest are simple grains in the form of baby cereals. Baby cereal comes premixed or in "flakes," and you add water or formula to it. Three different kinds are available: rice, barley, and oatmeal. Rice cereal is one of the easiest foods to digest. You can also find "health food" versions of baby cereal that are made with brown rice or whole oats. As long as these are intended for feeding babies, you can choose this option.

Follow directions on the cereal package and make sure you don't *under*constitute: That means if the instructions tell you to put 1/4 of a cup of water in, don't put 1/8 of a cup of water, thinking that if it's thicker, it'll be better. (On the other hand, you can put in *more* water if your child is not yet used to the consistency, and her tongue is sticking a little on the food.) To repeat: Never add *less* water than the manufacturer's instructions suggest.

Never add less *water to the cereal than the manufacturer's instructions suggest.*

Occasionally you will find cereal in jarred form. Use it if you like, but you are probably going to throw away a lot of the leftovers.

Introduce wheat cereals last. There are good reasons to delay adding wheat to children's diets, even until age two, for children with family histories of specific wheat allergies or strong tendencies toward asthma and eczema.

Wheat warning: Many commercial baby cereals that are labeled "mixed cereal" contain wheat. Instead of saying "wheat" right on the box, however, as they would for "rice cereal," "barley cereal," and "oatmeal cereal," the box that has wheat in it says "mixed cereal." It doesn't mention wheat at all! Introduce wheat only after you've introduced the other three grains. Once you get around to introducing wheat into your child's diet, which should happen at eight months, you can also give her tiny pieces of pasta that she can scoop up to feed herself.

> Warning: Never feed your child directly from the food jar unless you know she will finish it. When you put a spoon from mouth to jar, you introduce bacteria from your child's mouth into the jar. Once the jar is closed, you have created a great germ-growing factory. You run the risk of giving your infant food poisoning when you feed her with it the next time.

Fruits and vegetables

Once baby has tried cereal successfully, you may add fruits and vegetables. Because texture is important for your child to learn about, offer a real banana when your baby is about eight months old. Instead of puréeing it in a blender or buying a jarred version, mash a ripe one with a fork and let your baby scoop it up with her hands to eat. Avocado is another good choice for this technique, and it's a vegetable to boot!

It is easier for baby (or anybody) to digest yellow vegetables than green ones. With that fact in mind, introduce your baby to carrots, squashes, and sweet potatoes first. Don't include corn, which is one of the hardest foods to digest. Don't worry if your child turns a little yellow on the tip of her nose and cheeks after eating lots of yellow veggies. It's not jaundice. It's

About Fruit Juices

Fruit juice is not a good substitute for real fruit, nor is it a source of good nutrition. Fruit juice is little more than sugar water, and it can cause diarrhea and tooth decay. Freshly squeezed fruit juice is too thick for infants to digest, so even a juicer won't make a good food out of fruit for your infant.

The rule is *no juice* until after age two (with a few exceptions for managing constipation or at the doctor's instruction).

from carotene, a naturally yellow, vitamin-rich substance in the vegetables, and it's good for baby. The color eventually fades.

Wait to introduce citrus fruits and berries until after ten months, because these too can be hard for baby to digest and may trigger allergies in some children.

Protein

You can start to add protein foods at seven or eight months. That includes soft cheeses, yogurts, tofu, poultry, and beans. Go very slowly with each new protein because they are hard for baby to digest and often require some chewing besides. If you are choosing a vegetarian lifestyle, be aware of special considerations for providing B_{12} and iron. For details, see the Vegetarian Food Pyramid in Chapter 10 (page 133).

Do not start red meat or fish yet. Early introduction of red meat has been linked to development of colon disorders in adult life. Fish—and, in particular, shellfish—allergies are common. These problems are less likely to occur if you wait until baby is almost age two to introduce him to fish and red meats. Peanut butter should also be avoided until age two.

Egg whites are pure protein, but don't introduce them to your baby until after the first birthday. However, you may add egg yolk to the diet at six months—but only in hard-boiled form. Before children reach age two, cholesterol from eggs is OK for them, with rare exceptions in cases of families with inherited cholesterol disorders. Ask your doctor to guide you. The majority of six-month-old children can eat as much egg yolk as they like. (By age two, a baby should be cut back to about three egg yolks a week.)

~

Warning: Bad Reactions

Stop feeding immediately if your child

- vomits,
- has explosive diarrhea—particularly with blood in it,
- develops a significant rash, or
- develops swollen eyes or lips.

Call your doctor if any of these symptoms occur and, again, stop feeding immediately. Give water and wash your child's hands and face gently and thoroughly. Your doctor will help you figure out whether your child is allergic to the food before you try any other new foods.

Allergies

An allergy is the response of your body to something it doesn't want in your body. The body creates antibodies to "foreign" things in the system, and that antibody stays in the memory of your immune system to fight off future attacks by the same kinds of organisms. In some cases, we keep that memory forever; in others, only for a few years. The body's allergic response can be violent, causing air passages to swell so that breathing is very difficult. It can even lead to death if left untreated. Fortunately, the majority of allergic reactions are limited to itchy, runny eyes and nose and maybe a scratchy feeling in the throat.

Most food allergies start in the first year of life. In fact, the earlier you introduce foods, the more likely and the more severe allergies can be. That is why you are advised to wait until your child is a bit older—closer to one year old—before offering such foods as egg white, citrus fruits, and berries.

Many kids have "skin allergies"; that is, they break out in eczema when exposed to certain triggers. Some of those kids are

~

"Do I breast-feed (or bottle-feed) my baby before the meal or after the meal?"

Offer your hungry baby the breast (or bottle) first, and after a few sucks introduce the new foods. Be careful not to let her fill up entirely on milk or she will have no room for the new solid food. After solids, again offer the breast or the bottle or, even better, a cup of water, because she may be thirsty after the meal. Water is especially good because it washes out the baby's mouth after solids. Giving the water afterward is a great way to avoid cavities and tooth decay once your baby develops teeth.

On the other hand, if your child is not particularly ravenous but is interested in the food that's on the table, there is no reason you absolutely must give milk first. You have to "go with the flow," so to speak. By the time they are a year old, many children have weaned themselves to about half the amount of milk they took before starting solids.

also likely to be asthmatic. Often children with asthma and
eczema are also allergic to foods including milk protein, wheat,
peanuts, egg whites, berries, and citrus fruits. These are the
usual culprits, but the suspect list may be even longer. Your
child may benefit from a full allergy evaluation if he fits the
classic picture of asthma, eczema, and allergies.

Sometimes a blood test can be done to decide whether a child
is allergic to a food. Other times the description of symptoms is
sufficient to conclude that there is an allergy. The younger the
child, the less accurate blood testing is for allergies, however.
Allergies are often overdiagnosed.

Note: If you or family members are allergic to a specific food,
you are best off avoiding it during pregnancy as well.

How Much Food Does My Baby Need?

Once your infant has learned the logistics of eating solid foods,
you will have to learn to deal with your baby's own opinions
and appetites. Like you, she will not always be hungry to the
same degree, and one day's beloved peas may be another day's
food reject.

Although sometimes it seems your baby can't wait for the
next spoonful, never shove food into your baby's mouth. When
your baby has had enough, she will usually let you know just by
not opening her mouth. But it is also possible that she just needs
a minute and some breathing room before eating a little more.
Offer another spoonful at least once after she has signaled
disinterest. If she "tells" you "no, thank you" again, take her
seriously and put away the food, regardless of how little she has
eaten. There is always the next meal, and the invaluable lesson
learned by your infant is to pay attention to her own signals of
hunger or fullness. By the same token, when your little

"energizer" keeps on going, offer another serving even if *you* think she has had enough. It's *her* job to decide how much she needs to eat on any given occasion.

Home-Made Baby Food

If you choose to make your own baby food, buy the jarred versions of different foods first, so you can see how runny it's supposed to be. It's the best way to judge food consistency, because these commercial products have been made after extensive research by nutritionists and developmental experts. To start with, everything you feed baby has to be in puréed form, particularly before teeth arrive. By the time children are about eight to ten months, you may offer thicker food. Commercial baby foods are "staged" to take into account the child's developmental and chewing ability. Staged foods are typically labeled as "First Foods," "Stage 2," "Stage 3," and so on.

Make food in your blender and then pour it into ice cube trays to freeze for later. Pop out one cube at a time from the tray to feed baby. A typical ice cube happens to be the approximate serving size of food for a child between the ages of six and ten months. Thaw the food in the refrigerator, if time permits, or in a small saucepan while stirring. Avoid microwaving because it tends to leave both hot and cold "spots" in the food.

Baby Wants a Cracker?

Parents often ask me about whether crackers and teething biscuits are good to give their teething baby. Babies should teethe on teethers and eat crackers. It is very easy to choke on a so-called teething biscuit, and I strongly recommend *not* using food for this purpose. When your child is teething, give him appropriate objects to teethe on, things that don't pose a choking hazard. Soft biscuits or crackers can be fun for your older infant to eat, once the first two teeth break through, especially if you let him hold one in each hand.

> Dear Dr. Paula,
>
> Joey, nine months old, is starting to drink out of a sippy cup. As for finger foods, he occasionally gets down a Cheerio, but otherwise he sticks to jarred foods. He gags when I try to give him anything else, so that tells me he is not ready yet. My older son was this way also at Joey's age. By the way, Joey is still toothless.
>
> Joey's mom

> *Dear Joey's mom,*
>
> *Joey is a typical older infant. He still takes a bottle but can also use a sippy cup. His gag reflex is still very "alert." You correctly recall that your older son used to gag on solids too, and clearly that is no longer an issue for him. Somewhere between infancy and toddlerhood, the swallow reflex "learns" to calm down. Keep offering a combination of lumpy jarred foods and safe finger food choices.*

Feed "Myself"!

Around the tenth month is the wonderful time when children start to feed themselves. This is not a time to teach table manners! It is a *good* thing when a ten-month-old child puts her fingers in food—that is how she learns about texture, smell, and

First Finger Foods

- Fruit shavings
- Thin cheese strips
- Chopped hard-boiled egg
- Soft banana
- Soft, baked "french fries"
- "Tea" sandwiches: crustless, soft bread lightly spread with vegetable purée

taste. By all means, let your child dip her fingers into the food to feed herself. Don't discourage it. It is part of the normal development process and essential to it. These older infants also start to manage "finger foods." These are the foods that baby can actually hold and not just dip a hand into. After the first birthday, hard-scrambled eggs are a great finger food.

Let baby hold utensils

Put a spoon in each hand once your baby reaches about eight months. The brain needs to do something with both hands simultaneously at that point, so the child will be more capable and successful with whatever he is trying to do. Apparently this helps to develop coordination. Your baby may not succeed right away; learning to feed yourself takes time. Use a soft-edged spoon with an angled handle, designed for small hands to aim easily at the mouth.

After six months, start to encourage your baby to hold his own bottle and introduce a cup with two handles and a sippy top (if you haven't guessed, this is a lid that baby can sip from). Wonderful sippy cups are available, including types that don't spill. Let your child start to learn how to sip from a cup just by putting one in front of him. Here's a good tip: Don't offer a bottle at the high chair at all, only a sippy cup. Help your growing child separate the "sucking for comfort" message from the "drinking for thirst" concept.

No-Nos When Feeding Solids

Don't season food

Adults will often judge their baby's food by whether they would like to eat it themselves. However, children like bland food, so there is no reason to add spices. When you taste your baby's food, you may think it has no taste. That's not true for the child whose taste buds are just developing and in fact are probably very sensitive to the new tastes and textures that you're presenting. Spices can also induce allergic reactions.

Don't add sugar to food

There is no reason to sweeten baby's food. Commercially made food is more likely to be sugar-free now than in the past. But if you're thinking, why not add a little sugar, think again. Sugar already exists naturally in all foods. Extra sugar only stimulates the pancreas to produce excessive insulin, which is unnatural and may lead to sugar intolerance later. Excess sugar is also bad for teeth and can cause diarrhea.

If you make baby food, never add salt

Too much salt is very difficult for an infant's kidneys to handle and can even cause serious problems.

Avoid feeding juice

There's no place for juice in your child's diet, unless your doctor specifically advises you to use juice to help a child who has hard stools (constipation).

No fat-free foods for babies

Parents often ask me about low-fat diets for babies. I always tell them that it's *good* for babies to look chubby. Parents seem to think babies should be on low-fat yogurt or low-fat cheeses or foods prepared with Pam cooking spray instead of butter. No. Babies need fats for the development of the nervous system. The fat found in whole milk is good for your baby. So don't ever put your child on a low-fat diet. If there is family history for early coronary disease, there may be some modifications to this rule, but only in extreme circumstances; your pediatrician will guide you.

Three Meals a Day?

Does it matter what your child eats for breakfast versus dinner, or how much your child eats at any time of day? The answer is no, it doesn't matter. Your baby isn't going off to work, so loading of food at the top of the day is not necessary. Don't expect your child to down three meals a day, either. Your baby is growing all the time and is likely to want to eat something throughout the day, not just at those times when you are ready to sit down for breakfast, lunch, or dinner.

> A typical diet at about eight months is cereal and fruit for breakfast, yogurt and a vegetable for lunch, maybe with an egg yolk, and a little poultry and a vegetable or a fruit for dinner. Somewhere in between you may offer another fruit or cereal.

Feed on demand

I have parents who worry that their babies will become overeaters, obese, or constant snackers if they are fed on demand, but that's not the case. It is best for your infant to eat small, frequent meals. Parents are often confused about what's a meal and what's a snack. They'll ask, how many meals a day and how many snacks a day? Let me reassure you: There is no way to tell meals and snacks apart at this age, especially if you are offering only healthy foods choices. The key is not to think in terms of meals and snacks at all. Just think in terms of good nutrition and healthy food habits whenever food is served.

Dear Dr. Paula,

I wonder if my ten-month-old Brianna is getting enough variety in her diet. These are the only foods she eats: bananas, yogurt, crackers, bread, pancakes, and a little scrambled egg and cheese. I have tried all kinds of fruits and vegetables, and she won't eat them. What is your opinion? (She is breast-fed twice a day as well.) Thanks.

Brianna's mom

Dear Brianna's mom,

Congratulations! Your child is doing great. She eats a sufficient variety of foods to grow strong and healthy, even without the vegetables, although you can continue to place small finger-food veggies on her plate in case she changes her mind. Don't discount the value of the twice-a-day breast-feeding—that adds to your baby's good nutrition.

4

Infant Roadblocks

Dear Dr. Paula,

My nine-month-old, Max, is having trouble with solids. He was doing fine until one day. Then he started to cry as soon as he saw the baby food come out. For some reason he won't take any, and he cries and cries until I give him his bottle, and then he wolfs it down like he's starving! After that he won't take any solids, even if I offer him the fruits he used to like so much. Did I do something wrong or is something wrong with Max's swallowing? I'm really worried. Thank you for your help.

Laura, Max's mom

Dear Max's mom,

It sounds like Max is very hungry and is showing his preference for the bottle. That's normal. He wants that bottle, and then, of course, he isn't hungry anymore after finishing the whole 8 ounces. I would try giving him his bottle before he starts to cry but only fill it up halfway. Then while he is sitting in his

*high chair, happily sucking, I would bring out the
pears and let him dig in. I would even let him play
with it until he feels it's "friendly" again. If things go
well, you can also offer him the rest of the bottle after
he's eaten some solids, just to wash it down. He may
not want more milk at that point, but that's OK. He
is supposed to start weaning from formula about now
anyway. Avoid making the mistake of thinking he still
needs to get 32 ounces a day so you don't hinder the
process of moving on to more solid food. Good luck.*

Parents are sometimes surprised that feeding problems can start
this early in their child's life. Parents may perceive the first year
as being relatively easy when it comes to feeding. When people
think about feeding problems, they think of picky eaters and
toddlers. Infancy seems to be a blissful period in terms of
feeding. In fact, a lot can go wrong, despite the best intentions.

Problems roughly fall into two categories—those that are
psychologically based and those that are more physically based.
They overlap, and one can lead to the other.

Psychological Problems with Feeding

Well-meaning parents usually create these problems.

Feeding to please

That's the mother or father who's smiling, who's playing
airplane with a spoon to get the child to eat. The child is
eating *only* to get a smile. The child may not even be hungry.
(See commandments 1 and 2 in Chapter 1, pages 5 and
6.)

Parents who delay introduction of food

A parent may delay the introduction of food because he or she is afraid baby is going to choke, so the parent never really presents lumpier textures. The anxious parent leaps excitedly to "rescue" an infant who is merely learning how to put her tongue around a bit of lumpy food. This child doesn't get the chance to learn what to do with chunky food as opposed to puréed food. Parents who delay giving children "real" foods are causing their infants to miss an important developmental opportunity.

Parents who "push" baby to drink too much milk

Baby gets all of his hunger satisfied by large quantities of milk. This is often because the parents are afraid to watch the child struggle with the task of learning how to eat solid food. This child learns to crave the bottle and to lean on it for comfort and security long after he needs it for nutrition.

Physical Problems with Feeding

Food intolerances

At under one year of age, your infant can have unrecognized food intolerances. A baby who is cranky a lot of the time may be in pain from intolerance to certain foods even at this young age. (Teething is often blamed mistakenly for *all* crankiness.) Often parents and doctors overlook this possibility and look for other explanations for the irritability. You can help figure it out by watching to see if your infant becomes especially cranky after eating certain foods. Then you can try to eliminate those foods. Withhold that food for a period of time, usually at least a week. Never remove more than one food at a time, or you'll never know which food may be causing the problem. Watch for a difference. Then give the suspected food back and observe again. If there's a relapse of discomfort in your child you can conclude that the food was to blame. At this point, contact baby's doctor.

Lactose intolerance.   Infants who are lactose intolerant may be unhappy, cranky, and in pain. Lactose intolerance will make an infant bloated and gassy. They are also learning to dislike food. (That's how a physical problem can lead to a psychological one.) There are children who are loath to eat because they are accustomed to being in pain when they eat.

Food allergies.   Even infants can develop food allergies. Allergies can also contribute to the early appearance of eczema and asthma. Milk, peanuts, and egg whites, in particular, are common causes of allergies. That's why you should add foods slowly, one at a time and in a specific order.

Eczema

Scaly, itchy skin can be a symptom of an allergy to cow-milk protein. You may also be feeding a future asthmatic because eczema and asthma are often twin curses. Recognize it as food-related and you may be able to put off or dampen these medical conditions.

Overfeeding

Parents always ask: Is it possible to overfeed an infant?

The answer is yes. Adding cereal to the bottle contributes to obesity. You can also overfeed an infant even plain formula by trying too hard to encourage your child to eat.

You can also overfeed a breast-fed infant, even though it's generally thought that you can't because the baby controls the flow. But if you force your nipple into the baby's mouth at every cry, that develops into a bad habit. I've had mothers say, "My baby is hungry all the time," and I ask, "How do you know?" They answer, "Because whenever I put him on my breast, he sucks." The fact is that he even sucked on his thumb in utero. That's not proof that your child is hungry. That's proof that babies suck. It's a reflex.

Feeding to soothe

A parent who always offers food when their infant cries is teaching that baby to solve every problem with food. Parents sometimes just don't know what else they can do to soothe a crying baby and the truth is sucking does work. Sucking releases brain endorphins, which are hormones that make you feel good. But your baby can suck on a thumb or a pacifier instead and have the same comforting result. You can even give him a diaper cloth to suck on, and it too will work just as well.

Overeating

An overeating baby takes in more calories than is required for growth and development. Newborns typically gain between one and two pounds a month. An overeater may gain four or five pounds a month. Some are genetically "programmed" to be large babies. They eat huge amounts of food and are incredibly happy and active. Without a family history of obesity, these infants will grow up healthy and strong and probably not even be overweight.

The other kind of overeating comes from parents who want a chubby baby because they think chubby equals healthy. These parents will do almost anything to keep the baby eating. Parents accomplish that by smiling broadly with every swallow and saying, "Mommy loves you," and planting a kiss on the forehead with every suck. That child will eat more because she has been conditioned to. Some parents may also be unable to tolerate their child's cry and will use food or the bottle or the breast for every tear. Infants learn quickly to eat to soothe themselves or their parents.

Needless to say, never force-feed or be aggressive with food. Eventually an infant will do one of two things: He gives up resisting and starts sucking, or falls asleep and rejects food altogether.

Underfeeding

Insufficient milk syndrome

When a baby isn't gaining weight, consider: Is baby getting enough milk? When you are formula-feeding, you can count the ounces he takes. You can't measure the ounces taken from the breast. Women who are not providing sufficient milk for their baby are often depressed and defensive about it—and sometimes totally unaware that the child could be underfed. An infant who gets insufficient nutrition in the first months of life will lag behind in milestones. Permanent fine-motor-skill deficits and learning disabilities have both been linked to early food deprivation.

How will you know? You need to monitor how much stool and pee your baby is producing. Breast-fed babies may poop with every feeding, although there is a lot of variability. (If your baby is one of those who are gaining weight and seem perfectly healthy but don't seem to poop more than once every few days, don't worry about it.) The usual pattern is eat, pee, poop, gain weight. A baby who isn't getting enough will fail somewhere in that chain. You may not pick it up at the "eat" point, especially if you are breast-feeding, but hopefully you'll recognize that she is not peeing enough. Diapers should be wet often, about six times a day in the first six months. The other clue is a cranky baby who is not comforted after eating or a listless baby who doesn't perk up during a feed. *Beware:* If your newborn is sleeping for long periods, you may initially feel "blessed," but it may be because he's actually too weak to wake up.

Undereating

There are infants who don't eat much because they were born prematurely and may feed very slowly, even burning more calories in the effort to feed than they actually receive. They take more time than other babies do to muster up the instinct to feed. Any baby who falls into this category needs careful medical supervision and a strict feeding plan.

Switching from Breast-Feeding to Bottle-Feeding

The American Academy of Pediatrics recommends that mothers breast-feed their babies exclusively for at least the first six

~

Failure to Thrive (FTT)

Failure to thrive can be caused by diseases, disorders, or metabolic problems. The most common medical reason for failure to thrive is undetected heart disease. Sometimes FTT is the result of an anxious parent feeding their child in some dysfunctional way. The infant may respond by clamping their mouth shut and turning away from food. This situation always requires medical intervention.

months. However, we live in a society where mothers often plan not to breast-feed for the whole year or for even the first six months. Often they haven't planned how to make the change to a bottle, and they run into difficulties. A breast-feeding baby is often reluctant to switch to a bottle nipple even after only a few months on the breast.

If you know in advance that you are going to switch to formula, make that introduction to the bottle early (even if it has breast milk in it). Add a bottle at least every other day as an insurance policy. You need to know that your child can be soothed and comforted by someone else.

Sucking on a bottle nipple is different than sucking on a breast. However, the manufacturers of nipples work very hard to replicate the action of the breast in the design of their nipples.

Dear Dr. Paula,

I finally did it! I've managed to successfully combine breast-feeding and going back to work. Michael, my four-month-old, wasn't too thrilled at first, but little by little he is learning to take my expressed breast milk by bottle when I'm not home. Pumping at work is actually a welcome "coffee break." No one has given me a hard time. Once Michael gets a few ounces of my milk, he moves over pretty easily to a few ounces of formula. And when I do breast-feed after I come home, it's fine because he's not cranky. And I'm not so stressed out by the whole feeding thing. Thank you. I couldn't have done it without your guidance.

Michael's mom

Dear Michael's mom,

YOU are the one who did it. Great going! Sometimes only "fear of failure" gets in the way. Soon you can look forward to giving Michael cereal and then applesauce. That's when the fun begins!

Gerber has created a fabulous new silicone nipple. It's very flexible. When an infant sucks on it, it extends like a human nipple and then retracts again. The company claims if you use this nipple from the very beginning to supplement breast-feeding, your baby won't experience nipple confusion and will continue to feed happily, switching back and forth between breast and bottle.

The Infant Who Gags

Some infants gag and choke on food when they start "solids." You must report this occurrence to your doctor. Some infants choke on puréed foods, and the doctor needs to rule out any anatomical problems such as a blocked or narrowed larynx (throat) or a poorly coordinated swallow mechanism.

Once it's established that there is no physical problem, there are other causes to consider. Gagging on solid food is sometimes a baby's way of saying "I don't like this," or even "I'm allergic or intolerant to this food." So don't persist in offering the same food.

Sometimes a parent will confuse ordinary development of the gag reflex with a dangerous choking episode. The baby gags a little, and the parent becomes alarmed and goes back to feeding formula. When the parent panics, the baby is also scared and may refuse to eat any textured food. The baby doesn't get all her nutritional requirements met. My best advice is: Calm down. We have a gag reflex for a reason; it prevents large pieces of food from getting lodged in our throats. It's protective. Of course, frequent choking episodes require medical attention.

~

"My six-month-old has me worried. She won't eat anything. I have tried cereals and fruits and veggies, but she just gags and spits it out. She takes the bottle just fine and is gaining weight. Why won't she eat?"

Some babies just aren't ready when you are. Stop offering solids for a week and then try again. Avoid getting worked up about the timetable and let nature take its course. I promise, all healthy babies learn to eat!

Babies Who Spit Up

All babies spit up, which is why there are spit-up cloths. There is a difference between spitting up and throwing up. You need to make sure your baby doesn't have a medical condition like reflux. (It's technically referred to as GERD: gastro-esophogeal reflux disorder.) With reflux, the food doesn't stay in the stomach; it comes back up. And it may come back up almost in its entirety.

This condition leads to discomfort and sometimes weight loss and is usually treated with medication. Severe reflux, if untreated, can even lead to asthma and wheezing. Children who have reflux and wheeze often stop wheezing if treated for their reflux. However, it is often overdiagnosed. Most infants who spit up are quite happy and gain weight. These infants do not need medications. Just bibs.

Your doctor may recommend a change in feeding style. This is probably the only time your doctor may tell you to put cereal in the bottle to "hold the milk down." Putting cereal in the bottle is an unproven treatment, but some parents and doctors swear by it. It is also best to feed your infant in a semi-upright position. Your baby should be feeding at least at a 30-degree angle (see the illustration on page 24). And by the time the baby gets to solids she should be completely sitting up.

The Messy Child

When your baby is given solids she should be allowed to play with her food. Messiness is really a problem parents have, not babies! But it can lead to feeding problems later on if a heavy hand is used to keep an infant from touching his food. There are exceptions of course. If your infant is trying to say to you, "I am done eating," and now he is just throwing food around, take the hint. Remove it. But if your child is actually eating, let him be.

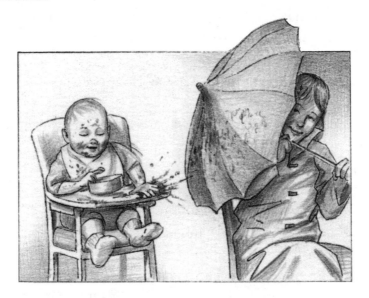

At the six-month visit I always tell parents to make sure to have a camera ready and to wear a raincoat when starting solid foods. They always look at me quizzically, and I say, "Trust me," and smile knowingly.

5

Toddlers

Dear Dr. Paula,

I have a thirteen-month-old son who is now on normal food and jarred baby food. It's been about three weeks, and I'm a little concerned that he's not eating enough. The only fruit he likes is applesauce. Sometimes he'll eat fruit cocktail, but only about five to ten pieces of fruit and then he spits some out. I've tried putting peaches or pears in a blender, but he still spits it out. I've tried pastas with sauce, and he spits that out, too. The only thing he really likes is any kind of vegetable. If I do try a new food, like macaroni or chicken and rice, some days he'll eat some of it, and others he won't touch it. Is this normal? Help!

Jack's mom

Dear Jack's mom,

Welcome to toddlerhood! I always tell parents that the challenging "twos" begin at one and end at three if you are lucky. Your thirteen-month-old is right on schedule. It will help you cope if you understand that

> *his nutritional needs, in terms of calories, has actually decreased at this age, and his growth will not even come close to matching his first year's growth rate for several more years. However, as "normal" as your son is, avoid pitfalls such as offering sugary foods to inspire his appetite. (Buy fruit cocktail in water or rinse off the heavily sugared juice before serving.) Expect his intake to look good to you only when viewed from an "every three days" perspective. It's a good thing to move on to finger foods and away from jarred. How nice that he actually likes vegetables. (I would get video proof of this to show him later if I were you!)*

A toddler is someone who can "toddle," which generally means someone above the age of nine or ten months who has just started to walk. This stage lasts until about thirty months. Your toddler is really much more interested in "toddling" than in eating. This is the time children are climbing, running, jumping, and getting into things, becoming more skilled each day—with little interest in slowing down for food.

It's also important to understand that toddlers' favorite word is "no," and their favorite expression is "I do it myself!" That's the key to unlocking the mysteries about toddlers and food. With these few vital facts in mind, a parent has a better chance of surviving the tempestuous toddler years.

Rule Number 1:
Toddlers Grow Less Than Infants

Toddlers don't grow as rapidly or evenly as infants do. This can worry parents. Not seeing much change in their child's height and weight can undermine a parent's confidence.

Psychologically and developmentally toddlers are in a stage of seeking independence. In the first year, it was easy to see if you were a "good" parent by those monthly visits where the baby gained weight and grew. That situation changes in the toddler years.

Here's the scene: Mom comes in to the pediatrician with her twenty-one-month-old son and sees that he has grown only half an inch and gained one pound in six months. She was worried even *before* her baby was measured because she sees that her child isn't eating very much. I try, even at the ten-month visit, to prepare parents for this upcoming period by telling them that in the next few months they are going to see a real slowdown in the amount of food their child eats. I take out the growth chart and show them how after ten months the growth line flattens in all three arenas: head, length, and weight. Not much growth happens in year two compared to year one. Rule 2 follows directly from Rule 1.

Rule Number 2:
Toddlers Do Not Eat as Much as Infants Do

The toddler is going through a stage of separation, and one way to become independent is to say "no." And so the child says "no" to almost everything. And the biggest no is to food. Luckily, because they don't grow much at this stage (see Rule 1), they don't *need* as much food as you think, either.

> Dear Dr. Paula,
>
> At my thirty-month-old son's play group, they keep daily reports on all the children. They have circled on Billy's sheet that he has unbalanced meals. As long as I send broccoli, mac and cheese, and applesauce every

day, I know he will eat it. He loves the stuff. I have failed in the school's eyes. Any advice?

                                        Billy's mom

Dear Billy's mom,

Sounds to me like Billy is doing just fine. In fact, his lunch is quite balanced. You need to have a talk with the school about this one. Billy should not be expected to eat balanced meals every day. Balance is something that improves with age. Toddlers often don't eat very much, and pressure from you or the teachers will only make him more reluctant. Let him be.

Your Terrific (Not Terrible!) Toddler

Children at this age love to play with finger paint, and they love to use their hands. Use your toddler's natural curiosity as an opportunity to enhance interest in food. This is the age to invite them into the kitchen to be little chefs and cook with you, even if it means

> FYI: The typical toddler needs to eat about 44 calories per pound of body weight per day.

letting them put their hands into food in order to create things. Encourage them as they make faces on their sandwiches, using a carrot stick here and an olive there for decoration. Let them use healthy foods along with your supervision, and these foods will remain in their consciousness, becoming a part of their expectations of what good foods are.

Kids in the kitchen.   Children enjoy helping in the kitchen and often are more willing to eat the foods they help prepare. Involve your child in planning and preparing some meals and snacks for the family. Give kitchen tasks that are age appropriate. Be patient.

Two-year-olds can perform the following tasks:

- wipe table tops
- snap green beans
- scrub vegetables
- wash salad greens
- tear lettuce
- play with utensils
- bring ingredients from one place to another
- break cauliflower

Tips for Feeding Toddlers

Make food available all day.   Food should be available all day long, within your child's easy reach, so that your child can choose food and pick it up as the urge directs. Toddlers are not going to eat three meals a day. However, your toddler will refuel; that's all food should be for.

Keep portions small.   Toddlers have small stomachs and short attention spans, so keep portions small. You don't want your toddler to feel that he is not pleasing you when he doesn't clean his plate, and you shouldn't feel that he failed if he did not finish. The temptation to play with food grows if a large amount is left on the child's plate. Think of a portion as the size of two walnuts.

Offer some slightly crunchier foods.   Toddlers usually have a lot more teeth than babies do. Although they still can't eat a raw carrot stick, they can certainly eat a slightly steamed one.

No running with food.   Make sure your children don't run with food in their hands. Try to have them eat in a sitting position or at least while standing still.

Experiment with new tastes.   Occasionally let your toddler try little bits of unusual-tasting food—not heavily herbed and spiced, but not so bland either. For example, many toddlers will taste olives and pickles, and that sets the stage for later appreciation.

Presentation is important.   Food should be colorful, especially vegetables, which are hard for kids to swallow. Because red is an "exciting" color to toddlers, offer red peppers instead of green. Try sweet potatoes. Naturally colorful foods are also often more nutritious.

Keep expectations realistic.   If you don't expect your toddler to eat a whole lot of his vegetables, then you won't be disappointed. You might try capitalizing on the little-known fact that toddlers will usually choose whatever option you mention *last*. Say "Would you like cake or broccoli?" not "Would you like broccoli or cake?" (If you are trying to get him to try broccoli!)

Model by sitting down and eating, even if your child doesn't. She might come over and climb up on your lap, and then there's a chance she may sample what you're eating. Do not eat standing at the kitchen counter if you are hoping to see good table manners down the road.

Eat what you want your child to eat.   Toddlers often imitate what adults do. Sometimes you can use this to get them to try new foods. Put a little food on *your own* plate that you would like your child to eat. Don't be surprised if your child eats it because "yours is always better."

Food jags are common at this age.   This is the common age for picky eating in general. Don't panic if your child eats the same two or three foods over and over. Always continue to offer other foods, but don't make a big deal out of it. One toddler in my practice will eat only white foods. Another has meatballs morning, noon, and night. These jags do not last forever. As long as your child jags on basically healthful food that you provide, go with the flow.

> Dear Dr. Paula,
>
> My two-year-old is driving me nuts! Either I cater to her, which encourages her pickiness, or I simply say, "Here is the meal, like it and eat it or be a little hungry." If I do the latter, then I am up in the night with a pitiful little one saying, "Eat, mommy, eat." My husband suggested that I not cater to her at lunch. I will provide a tasty well-balanced meal at lunchtime, which she will have the option of eating or not. For dinner, I will cater to her whims a bit more so she will not go to bed hungry.
>
> Katy's mom

> *Dear Katy's mom,*
>
> *Part of the toddler's "job," so to speak, is to deal with all the stimuli around them. Food is offered sometimes when they are not hungry and then exhaustion beckons them to sleep just when their tummy starts*

growling. I suggest not trying so hard to intervene in all these storms. Put out several food choices for her throughout the day and save the balanced meal concept for her preschool years. Overall she will sleep better, eat more, and, in the big picture, get a balanced diet over time. It's not the pickiness you need to avoid but the tantrums and misery she is attaching to food. Toddlers are picky; that's OK. She can eat the same healthful two foods for months and nothing bad will happen. If neither a fruit nor a vegetable crosses her lips, then be sure to give her a multivitamin hefty in vitamin C.

Dear Dr. Paula,

My twenty-two-month-old daughter rivals my culinary pickiness. Yesterday it was grits day, and she ate five bowls of grits all day—nothing else. Today was banana day, four jars of it, because she refuses to eat real bananas. I hope the bananas hold her all night.

Gretchen's mom

Dear Gretchen's mom,

Apples don't fall from pear trees. That's my way of pointing out that it's no surprise that mommy and toddler share the same food attitudes. Just remember that there are many ways to grow up healthy and strong. Your mom probably worried over you, too. Besides, grits and bananas for a few days is not so terrible. Try to have Gretchen see how well you eat now, so she can also learn from your good food habits.

Expect your toddler to be fussy.   He may want his sandwich cut a certain way. Go with it at this age. Let him help cut the food into his favorite shape. When he visits grandma and she doesn't have his special star-shaped cookie cutter, he will more readily tolerate the disappointment than he would back home with you. Trust me on this one. This is also the age where kids sometimes don't like it when the food on the plate "touches" other food. Just offer him a tray with compartments.

Get rid of the high chair. It's great for an infant who can sit but can't climb out. It's not so great for a toddler who can climb out and tip it over. Most healthy toddlers can easily get out of any high chair.

Eating and snacking are two sides of the same coin. To a toddler, there is no difference between eating and snacking. It's not important to distinguish between snacks and food. And if what you offer as a snack is really just junk food, that is *not* the message you want to teach.

Don't call attention to desserts. When you present several small servings of different foods, one might fall into the dessert category. Your toddler shouldn't be taught that there is a difference between dessert and other foods, because that only encourages food conflicts. In fact, a spoon of sweeter food, like applesauce, may be just the thing to stimulate the toddler's appetite for the rest of the meal. Everything that you offer your toddler should be food you would be proud to offer if there was a pediatrician at the table.

Don't bother taking your toddler to a restaurant. It's not fun for the toddler, and it's not fun for the parent. It certainly isn't fun for the wait staff and other customers, and your child's self-esteem doesn't need to be put to this social test. Toddlers do not have a good time when they are restrained in any way.

> **Dear Dr. Paula,**
>
> **Yesterday my picky eater ate broccoli. I could hardly believe it myself, but she managed to eat two bites of the "little green trees." She was rewarded with vanilla ice cream. She was told no ice cream unless she ate two bites of broccoli, so she decided to eat it. I tried not to make too big a deal out of it, knowing that if I did, she would certainly never repeat the performance.**
>
> Beth's mom

> *Dear Beth's mom,*
>
> *Here we see illustrated a seemingly logical system of reward (ice cream) in exchange for "good" behavior (eating broccoli). This is tempting, but be aware that this can backfire; the toddler is learning how to control you and her world through what she will or will not eat. You may be worried about calcium intake, but it would be just as instructive if Beth could eat both the broccoli and the ice cream in any order she pleased as long as she ate some of both. She may have only one bite of broccoli, but the message would be less hot-wired. Even giving Beth ice cream after broccoli without stating the connection would be better than encouraging the manipulative use of food.*

Outside Influences

Be on top of the situation even when your children are not with you. Some toddlers go to day care or to play groups or have play "dates." Look for settings that foster similar views to your own regarding food. If you are teaching your child not to crave candy, it is not helpful if every day at gym time she gets candy for climbing. Food issues tap into all of life's activities.

Dear Dr. Paula,

I awoke early in order to pack Steven's lunch for his first day at the day care center. I laughed as I tried to pack him a lunch, knowing what a challenge it is to get him to eat anything. I sent a jar of bananas, a jar of chicken sticks, a slice of American cheese, a plastic bag with some cheese crackers, and a snack cup of bran cereal. I figured surely he would eat something out of all of that. I know the child-care workers must have wondered what in the world mom was doing sending an almost two-year-old with jars of baby food, but you do what ya gotta do, right?

Steven's mom

Dear Steven's mom,

Now there's a creative effort! When sending your toddler off to others' care, it pays to include even foods he usually won't touch. It isn't necessarily a fairy tale when, at pickup time, the child-care worker tells you he ate all of it. Keep in mind how little a toddler's food behavior is based on appetite or hunger. Most of their food antics are only about attitude—theirs. And the goal is to keep presenting healthful foods. Steven's teachers will not balk at seeing the jar of baby food, but you might also send slices of fruit or a real banana in case he decides he is a "big boy" now when he is under the influence of his peers. Toddlers love to imitate others, and if his lunch mates are dipping fruit slices into applesauce, he might do the same.

~

Toddlers and Allergies

If your child has serious food allergies, I recommend that he not go to day care. If your child is allergic to peanuts, for example, which is a serious allergy, he is guaranteed to come across peanuts as an ingredient in many baked goods. Even with the best preparations and precautions, young children can come to serious harm in group circumstances when the staff is expected to respond to serious allergic reactions. As your toddler grows, his allergies may diminish or at least become less life-threatening. An older child can even look out for himself a bit and help to avoid the foods he is allergic to.

What *Do* Toddlers Need in Their Diets?

Calcium.   The essential missing piece in the diet could be calcium. Toddlers need a pint of milk a day or the equivalent. Although there is slower overall growth in the second year, toddlers' bones are still growing. Your child may go from being a "standard chubby" baby to a lanky preschooler.

Whole-milk products.   In the second year, children still need whole-milk products. Do *not* give your child nonfat milk or low-fat yogurt.

Fiber.   Toddlers are also busy learning how to use the toilet. They are often conflicted about whether to "let go" and make a poop. They may end up constipated. Add some fiber to their diet for assistance.

Extra fluids. Toddlers need extra fluid. It may not be easy to catch up with your toddler, but keep water handy. They don't need a constant flow, so avoid letting a bottle dangle from their mouths while they run around the playground.

Toddlers and Bottles

Most toddlers should be weaned from the bottle early in the toddlerhood period. From a nutritional point of view, that is one way to ensure that your child will not spend the entire toddler period drinking milk as his sole source of nutrition. This is a common pitfall. (Read all about it in the next chapter.) Sometimes a parent who is anxious because her child is disinterested in food is relieved when the child still drinks three or four bottles of milk a day. But that's a nutritional mistake. Your child could end up nutritionally depleted and anemic even if his weight continues to increase.

Breast-feeding toddlers usually wean themselves from the breast as their primary source of nutrition. They may just use it for occasional comfort in the second year. Nature has arranged for mother's milk to diminish in quantity and in sugar content after about a year's time. And that's a good thing, because it would be hard for your toddler to run and play attached to a breast!

For safety reasons, for proper speech development, and for visual coordination, a child should not have a bottle in his mouth all day. Children who do hold a bottle in their mouth talk with their teeth clenched around the nipple. In addition, once you get rid of the bottle, you will bring 650 milk calories down to about 320 calories of milk, which leaves room for hunger and increases the chances that your toddler will turn to other foods to satisfy it.

I also don't care for abrupt separation of baby and bottle. It should be done gradually early in toddlerhood, but matter-of-factly. Make an effort to spend long periods of time outdoors without a bottle. Your child is going to get thirsty, so give him the thrill of drinking from a sippy cup or a sports bottle. Toddlers enjoy squeezing the liquid into their mouths. Bring an extra change of clothes along, because getting wet is unavoidable at first.

The Toddler Rule of Survival: Pick Your Battles

Dear Dr. Paula,

I have been avoiding buying any cookies or junk food because when it is in the house, we have chaos. Bree will fall on the floor screaming for a cookie if she knows they are anywhere in the house. I bought some today because my family will be trickling in tomorrow, and I wanted to have some snacks for them. Sure enough, Bree had a tantrum when she demanded a cookie as her dinner was served. We held firm and resisted her negotiating tactics—"Pease, mommy, just one cookie." She said, "I am not happy." Bree had a true tantrum yesterday at Chuck E Cheese at lunch, where we met some friends. She fell to the floor kicking and screaming. I ended up scooping her up and carrying her out the door. Help!

Bree's mom

This letter opens the door to my favorite Toddler Golden Rule of Survival: Pick your battles. The typical two-year-old toddler period is full of opportunities to disagree and disappoint your toddler. The fewer times you have to witness a meltdown, the better for all of you. A tantrum is not easy on your toddler either—it leaves her drained and sometimes humiliated. At this stage, a cookie would not be my choice of where to draw the line. I would put out a cookie along with dinner to avoid the confrontation. Next time, don't even bring cookies into the house. Your relatives will learn to enjoy more healthful snacks.

6

Toddler Roadblocks

Dear Dr. Paula,

Jesse is giving me back all the grief I gave my parents
when I was his age. He is the epitome of a picky eater
and refuses to try anything new. He eats no fruits or
vegetables except bananas or apples in baby-food jars.
He also eats baby-food green beans. Those are his only
fruits and veggies. Occasionally, he will eat a bite of
meat. The one food item he can't live without is
shredded cheddar cheese. He begs for it for every meal
and every snack. The only other foods he will eat are
toast, pancakes, and rice. Needless to say, we still
shovel in baby-food jars of fruits and vegetables. This
is only successful if he is fully distracted. I guess Jesse is
following in my footsteps, as I consider my taste buds
to be very sensitive and my food repertoire extremely
limited. I'm your basic "meat and potatoes" guy.

Jesse's dad

Dear Jesse's dad,

*You may find this hard to believe, but Jesse eats just
fine for his age and should be praised for it in order to*

*avoid creating a self-fulfilling prophecy. If you keep
seeing yourself in Jesse, then Jesse will see himself that
way as well. Step back and don't worry so much. No
matter what, you shouldn't be shoveling in any food.
And never feed by distraction. There is too much
emotion connected to food here. Keep reminding
yourself what toddlerhood is all about—curiosity and
movement!*

What Can Go Wrong

I've had parents come to my office crying because their lives
have turned into one huge food fight with their toddler. In this
situation, parents need to remember what a toddler is all about.
Normal physical and developmental changes that occur between
infancy and toddlerhood will result in a need for *less* food and
certainly for *more independent* food attitudes.

A change in the toddler's interest in and intake of food

This is the most common thing that goes "wrong" with toddler
feeding; parents aren't prepared for the sudden change. The
parent may still push food, but the normal toddler just isn't
interested. At the first pressure to "eat, eat, eat," you get a
toddler who quite naturally becomes assertive and responds,
"No, no, no!" A toddler will eat only when he is really hungry.
If your toddler is by nature what I refer to as a "ruminator"—
an infant who took forever to finish a bottle and who stashed
the mashed potatoes away in his cheeks like a squirrel—you
may have an intensely picky eater on your hands. Especially
avoid nagging this type of child because it is in his temperament

to view food dispassionately. Your toddler's picky eating habit can develop out of the need to stop *your* insistence that he must eat.

Toddlers who aren't allowed to feed themselves

A parent who decides her toddler is still an infant is headed for trouble. Some parents continue to spoon-feed their toddlers instead of allowing the toddler to feed himself.

> *Recently I saw a three-and-a-half-year-old suffering from failure to thrive. Lauren hadn't eaten more than 600 calories a day in a very long time. In fact, she hadn't gained an ounce since she was eighteen months old. She has learned to use food refusal to manipulate her mother. At nine months, mother said, "My perfect baby became a monster." "Monster" meant she stopped wanting to breast-feed. This, of course, is normal behavior for an emerging toddler. A toddler's job is to separate. Mother tried instead to cradle her daughter even more closely. Mom feared that Lauren wouldn't get enough food to eat. Lauren learned that if she would just accept even one Cheerio, it would satisfy her mom. So she learned to graze inefficiently, just to get mother off her back. She never truly developed hunger. She actually eats all day, maybe one Cheerio every fifteen minutes or so; not nearly enough to grow, of course. Her mother is obsessed that Lauren will die of starvation. She certainly has reason to worry, but the solution will take a lot of change in their feeding interaction. I strongly recommended psychological intervention for this family.*

"Eating to please" problems

The opposite side of the same coin is the child who readily opens his mouth and eats *everything* in order to please the parent. *Obesity and failure to thrive come from the same beginning.* The more passive child will eat because he wants to please mommy, and he wants her to stop nagging. This child becomes an overeater. The path the toddler chooses depends on his or her personality.

Inaccurate expectations about toddlers

Some people see infants as immature grown-ups who should grow up faster. That belief could lead parents to expect their toddler to act like a preschooler. Often it is fathers and grandparents who fall into this trap. Moms, who spend hours with their toddler, understand that it is delusional to expect their child to eat with a fork and knife. But a grandparent who comes to visit may look at your toddler and announce, "You are raising a wild beast. When his father was eighteen months, he ate with good manners."

Not likely! Expect a toddler to be sassy and independent, unable to sit at a table and eat for more than a few minutes, if that, and relatively disinterested in food.

What to Do

Allow your toddler to experiment with new tastes and textures. Research evidence suggests that your child will be less likely to try different tastes and textures later on if he is not allowed to experiment now. This is also why you shouldn't allow your child to eat junk food at this age. It *is* the right age, however, to offer a variety of good, healthful food choices. Allow a toddler to have easy access to good food. Don't put too much on the plate, however, or you will invite food play.

A stubborn child can restrict his food intake if you become a maniac over what he eats and when. If you present only healthful choices, your child will eat what his body needs. He'll choose enough from among those healthy foods to satisfy his growth needs. But a parent who is a "nut" over this issue can actually push a child into a food disorder, even at this young age. I have seen it happen with kids who are chronically underweight and pasty-looking, and I've seen it with fat children as well.

If you present only healthful choices, your child will eat what his body needs.

Parents who are overly involved with their child's food intake take away the pleasure associated with eating. When that happens, a toddler stops trying new foods. Just the *sight* of food on a plate or the aroma of food can become a turnoff. If there is too much pressure on toddlers to eat, they may stop experimenting.

> No matter how much you want your toddler to eat, do not get into the bad habit of begging. You know: "Please, just one bite." "Mommy made this just for you." This is where whining begins—*yours first.* You whine at your toddler to eat. Then by the time he becomes a preschooler he has learned to whine back.

Dealing with the Dessert Monster

Dear Dr. Paula,

Today went on forever. I never thought my girls would go to bed. We took them to a Chinese buffet, which offered a little bit of everything. Abby ate pickles and lettuce, and Beth ate nothing. I mean nothing. She kept saying "um" for "gum," as she had seen a gumball machine on the way into the restaurant. We told her no gum, candy, or cookies unless she ate some dinner. She was determined not to eat. When we got home she rushed to the pantry and begged for cookies. We said no. We were able to distract her with the bedtime routine. Then Beth disappeared. She had slipped off into the pantry, grabbed the stepladder, climbed up and grabbed the chocolate cookies. She was stuffing them in her mouth as quickly as she could. She had even shut the door to the pantry in hopes of eluding the search for her. When my husband found her, she had a tantrum. He backed down with the concession that if she would drink a cup of milk she could have one cookie. She drank two sips and then asked for a cookie. She was told she had to drink all of her milk. Dad walked out of the pantry for a moment. When he came back Beth was pouring the milk out of her cup. Now what do we do?

Beth's mom and dad

Dear Beth's mom and dad,

Congratulations. You now have a full-fledged dessert monster living in your pantry, and it will not be easy to wish it away. Your clever two-year-old has learned to control her emotions with food-related behaviors. Your concerns for her nutrition have led her to food refusal, food sneakiness, and her own unique food-management style. My advice is to back off from using food as a reward or punishment. Put small amounts of dessert foods within her reach regardless of her prior food performance record, and let Beth de-stress from all the food-related pressures she is juggling before she develops a long-standing food disorder.

~

Banish the Monster!

After a big, nutritious meal, out comes the dessert to smiles and sometimes even applause. The trouble is that dessert has come to equal junk food. Even when that is not the case, anticipating a food reward makes the meal itself seem like a punishment by comparison. And yet many parents take it for granted that offering dessert will improve a child's food intake. *Wrong!* Offering a food reward creates a dessert-craving monster and one who is difficult to retrain. The solution: Whatever you think of as dessert should be one of the servings of the meal and not held out as an after-meal reward.

Bottles

Too much milk offered

Another problem I sometimes see is the toddler who hasn't given up the bottle. The mother has stopped trying to get the child to eat food and has settled instead for the notion that "as long as she is drinking, it's OK, especially if it's milk." That can lead to the child who is getting too many calories and who's got rotten teeth. This child may also wind up with a speech defect. A child can develop iron-deficiency anemia, and even malnutrition, from drinking too much milk, although she may be gaining weight. A bottle of milk just isn't complete nutrition for a toddler.

Too little milk offered

But, of course, your toddler does need *enough* milk. She can even develop rickets, a bone deficiency, if she doesn't get enough calcium and vitamin D. This can also result in nutritional dwarfism. Children need calcium to grow, and vitamin D to make the calcium usable. Fortified milk provides both.

All juiced up

Toddlers easily get hooked on juice or other sweet liquids, which is how they wind up with dental cavities. I have often seen children who have to have teeth removed because the parents let their toddler have endless bottles of juice. One father so feared his child wasn't getting enough calories that he continued offering juice even *after* the dental disaster.

Multivitamins

I don't normally recommend multivitamins. If I do, the parent is often on the edge of mania about it. I've had some mothers and fathers get really aggressive, admitting to literally shoving food into their child's mouth out of fear and frustration. If giving a multivitamin alleviates enough anxiety so that this kind of desperate behavior stops, I would gladly prescribe a vitamin.

Not long ago I was contacted by a concerned mother who needed a second opinion. She said, "What do I do with my twenty-one-month-old daughter who will not chew meats and vegetables? If she does eat them, she swallows them whole and then vomits. What is wrong?"

My first inclination as the consultant was to find something wrong physically. I considered ordering upper GI and swallowing studies. These are invasive procedures. Instead I asked, "Does your daughter speak well?" The response was, "Oh yes, she speaks, she sings." Then it hit me. This was a very anxious mother. Earlier when describing the problem she said, "But she will die if she doesn't eat meat and vegetables." She also confided that her regular pediatrician also told her to stop worrying because her child will get her nutritional needs met in all the other foods she eats. I asked, "What other foods does she eat?" Mom responded, "She eats grapes, yogurt with fruit. She chews up an apple when I peel it." This child had no trouble chewing the foods she wanted to eat. This mother was forcing foods on her child who was squirreling the food in her mouth and then spitting it back out without chewing, or just swallowing it whole. I advised, "I hear how concerned you are. You are worried that she doesn't get enough meat and vegetables. Your child needs you to stop sending the message that she must eat these foods. Don't even offer them for a while. What you can do to ensure that she gets some of this category of nutrition is to offer a multivitamin and occasionally purée fruits and vegetables into a soupy form."

Vitamin warning: Many multivitamins taste delicious and are shaped specifically to appeal to young children. If the vitamins contain iron, a child can actually get a serious overdose and will need hospital management. And don't make the mistake of thinking that if one is good, two must be better. That is never true. Treat vitamins like medicine. Put them high up on a shelf where a child can't reach them.

Dear Dr. Paula,

This morning was Rose's appointment for her two-year checkup. She's a tiny mite, measuring in at the fifth percentile in height (2 feet, 8 inches) and at the twentieth percentile for weight (23 pounds). We discussed her poor eating habits. Her doctor told me to try the Yummy Bear vitamins. Rose will not take chewable vitamins, and we have tried squirting Poly-vi-sol drops into her at night. That's less than pleasant. Her doctor said these new vitamins are so kid-friendly that he had to quit giving them to his own kids because they liked them so much there was a potential for overdose. I am going to check this out.

Rose's mom

Dear Rose's mom,

Rose is your typical toddler, full of spit and fire. What's interesting is that despite how fussy she is in her food choices, her twentieth-pecentile weight is more than adequate. Be forewarned, overdosage of vitamins, particularly ones containing iron or fat-soluble components such as vitamins A and E, can pose a major health hazard.

Dear Dr. Paula,

My son is too little, in the fifth percentile at his two-year checkup. And he's a lousy eater. Yet he runs with more energy than I can muster. You'd think he would beg for those sugary Flintstone vitamins, but they were a bust. He needs vitamins. Given his size, are there blood tests that can be ordered to see specifically what he is lacking? He's very bright and overly active, so I think he must be OK. But how does a kid live on six crackers, a pancake, and two sausage links a day?

Craig's mom

Dear Craig's mom,

You sound like you need a little encouragement, but you are on the right track about toddlers and food— they don't need much. As for blood tests, it is routine to check a child's complete blood count at about one year of age. If it shows anemia, further tests are done to assess iron supplies in the body. If your doctor has not yet ordered this test, I would ask for it, along with a test for lead, required in some states, but a good idea for all children at this age. Beyond this, ordinary blood tests will not tell you much. By the way, your son's diet is so typical—starch and protein—and not so bad. Just try a different brand of vitamins, and keep modeling by eating a healthful variety of foods in full view of your son.

"My Child Eats Nothing"

Very often a parent will tell me, "My child eats nothing, but she continues to grow." In these cases I quip, "Well, plants can survive on air and water, so I guess your child must be a begonia." Parents usually don't think that's funny. Children, in fact, aren't begonias, and they do need a certain amount of nutrition. So when a parent tells me that a child eats nothing, I look at the little living being in front of me. Then I suggest that the parent write down all the food she sees her child eat. *Every morsel.* Often the parent comes back and sheepishly reports,

"You know, I never realized that my child does eat this much, even though it doesn't look like much to me." The parent may also notice that the child consumed more junk food than she thought she was allowing. The junk food is taking the place of the nutrients the toddler really needs. (A three-day food intake inventory can be very useful.)

> Dear Dr. Paula,
>
> As you suggested, I kept a food diary on Dane for a few days. Oops. I guess he eats more than I thought.
>
> Dane's mom

MENUS

Dane: age 2 years, 10 months

Sunday

8:00 A.M.
- 1/2 jar banana baby food
- 1/2 jar sweet potatoes baby food
- 1 nut-grain-strawberry cereal bar
- watered down V-8 Splash juice

10:00 A.M.
- 2 teaspoons strawberry/banana yogurt
- 2 bites scrambled eggs
- 1/4 piece French toast
- 1 bite apple Danish
- milk

12:00 P.M.
- a few potato chips

3:00 P.M.
- 7 chips with beans/sour cream/cheese dip
- 1 slice pepperoni pizza
- watered-down V-8 Splash juice

7:30 P.M.

- 1/8 cup orzo
- Dr Pepper
- 1 whole bean-and-cheese burrito
- rice with tomatoes
- 1/2 cup noodles with cream cheese eaten off his aunt's plate

Monday

9:00 A.M.

- 1/4 cup orange juice
- water

10:45 A.M.

- 4 pizza wedges
- mixed fruit cup
- 1/2 bag Chee•tos snacks

12:10 P.M.

- 8 oz. apple juice
- small bag pretzels
- 1 bite of cookie

3:00 P.M.

- 3 chicken nuggets (baked)
- 2 french fries
- 1/2 ear corn (on cob)
- 4 crackers
- 4 cheddar cheese slices
- water

6:30 P.M.

- 1 stick string cheese

Tuesday

7:00 A.M.

- pineapple slice and half a cereal bar
- glass of milk

12:00 P.M. (in play group)
- Italian tuna-fish dish (tuna, vegetables, sauce)
- peach and applesauce
- apple slices with cinnamon
- pineapple slices
- glass of milk

Snack
- animal crackers
- milk

3:00 P.M. (at home)
- milk

6:30 P.M.
- hamburger with cheese and ketchup
- pickle spear
- cup of pudding
- V-8 vegetable juice

Before bed
- applesauce and milk

Dear Dane's mom,

Yes, Dane does get plenty of calories and good variety, even if some days are better than others. Over the three days, his diet balances out well. One tip: Keep an eye on the amount of salty and fatty foods just to be sure Dane still has "room" for the other food groups.

Be Careful: Toddlers May Try Nonfoods, Too

Normal infants and young toddlers will put almost anything in their mouths. They will chug detergents and munch on plant leaves if given the opportunity. Eventually they learn what is not good for them. But at this stage, safety is really an issue. Be especially careful of things that look like food but aren't. I'll never forget the time my son was in grandma's bathroom a little too long. When he came out, he was holding the remains of a bar of guest soap, colored, scented, and shaped just like chocolate candy. It even came in a little gold box with individual compartments to look like chocolate. And then there was the time my daughter broke a tooth biting into a wax pear from the centerpiece bowl on the dining room table. . . .

At this stage, safety is really an issue. Be especially careful of things that look like food but aren't.

Dangerous Foods

Foods with pits; popcorn

Although we are thrilled when they try new foods, toddlers are not yet competent enough to chew on an olive and dispose of the pit. A child with a handful of popcorn is a child who can easily choke. The number-one aspirated food is popcorn. It is so light that simple inhalation can float that popcorn into the back of the throat and down into the lungs. That's a very bad place for any food to end up, and it can be a serious medical emergency.

The number-one aspirated food is popcorn.

Hot food

Kids don't think about temperature. Never serve food steaming hot or serious burns can occur in the child's mouth and throat.

Watch out for popcorn, hot dogs (especially cut into circles), grapes, sourballs, fresh doughy bread, and chewing gum. Don't let a toddler grab a handful of small round foods.

Hard, chunky foods; foods served with toothpicks

Just because you have left puréed foods behind doesn't mean your toddler is necessarily ready for big wedges of hard apple or cheese. I had a family who "invited" their toddler to their office party. Soon after, I was treating the child in the emergency room—he had choked on a piece of cheese with the toothpick still stuck into it!

Heimlich Maneuver for Infants

Learn the Heimlich Maneuver for coping with choking incidents. The technique can be adapted to small-sized bodies. This information is a must for parents and child-care workers. No excuses! Courses are offered widely in most community centers or local health departments. (See box on facing page.)

The Heimlich Maneuver for Choking Infants

Lay the child down, face up, on a firm surface and kneel or stand at the victim's feet, or hold infant on your lap facing away from you.

Place the middle and index fingers of both your hands below his rib cage and above his navel.

Press into the victim's upper abdomen with a quick upward thrust; do not squeeze the rib cage. Be *very gentle*.

Repeat until object is expelled.

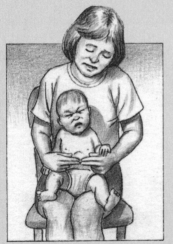 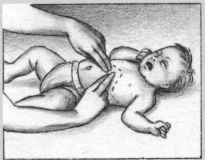

If the victim has not recovered, proceed with CPR. The victim should see a physician immediately after rescue.

Don't slap the victim's back. (This could make matters worse.)

7

Preschoolers

Dear Dr. Paula,

Jenny is now three years, four months old. She has
many food fads that come and go. The longest-
running favorite is her breakfast choice of pancakes,
which she asks for every single day. She eats mini
pancakes and a banana or cantaloupe. She will not eat
yogurt, eggs, or cereal (except dry Rice Krispies). The
only meat she will eat is a boiled ham sandwich or
chicken nuggets, but only from McDonald's. She also
loves quesadillas and grilled cheese sandwiches. Her
vegetable repertoire includes green beans, broccoli,
cooked carrots, and lettuce. She will eat most fruits,
but especially loves nectarines. She also loves
potatoes, rice, pizza, and dill pickles. Overall,
Mexican food seems to be her favorite. She wasn't
always good about trying new foods, but we have
never forced her to eat anything she didn't like. I
consider her to be a fairly good eater, and she even
manages to eat something from each food group
each day.

Jenny's mom

> *Dear Jenny's mom,*
>
> *Jenny couldn't be more typical of a young preschooler. The memory of past pickiness is already fading. You are offering appropriate opportunities for her to explore the food world without judging her by her past toddler performance. This is vital. Sometimes we lock into a negative opinion of our children's eating behavior, and it is hard to see the progress as they grow. Good job!*

As much as your two-year-old was an undisciplined wild bloom, your preschooler is almost the exact opposite. She is highly communicative and mostly cooperative and eager to mimic you for the purpose of being just like you. It's my favorite age. You can leave the house just holding her hand. No stroller. No diapers (some exceptions, of course). And she can eat very much like you eat.

Their safety "valve" is mostly in place—the way they swallow and chew is much more developed. This is a perfect time to teach some of the skills you have been chomping at the bit to get to—eating a sandwich or biting into a whole apple, for example.

Getting to Know Your Preschooler

What are the nutritional needs of a preschooler? There is a lot of physical growth between the ages of three and five that was temporarily put on hold during the toddler years. Between the ages of three and five, preschoolers suddenly are more like "little big people."

Previously I told you toddlers need to graze and need to have food always available. That's not necessary anymore. Your child is now bigger and can eat more food at one time. A preschooler is also less impulsive and has a longer attention span. Preschoolers can be expected to sit with food and use the time for more than just a "quickie fueling." A four-year-old can stop what he is doing because there is a meal coming. Dinner can include conversation and expectations on how to eat different foods. It's time to bring out the artichoke, for example. Kids are curious and will enjoy the "adventure" of trying new foods. Finally food is becoming more similar to what it is for adults— an opportunity for community, for sharing, for learning, and for feeling good inside.

The preschooler doesn't have as much emotion about food as the toddler does. The preschooler is less driven than was the toddler by the need to control what goes in and what comes out. You are reaching a stage where your child will eat what he likes and try a taste of what he doesn't like (assuming little pressure is put on him). Food will not be as limited in scope as it was during the toddler years.

This is the time to provide opportunities to eat a wide variety of foods. Even if your child doesn't like the artichoke, *you* can eat it and demonstrate the technique, and your child may consider trying one next time. Take your child to different ethnic restaurants. Food can even provide opportunities to teach charity.

This is the time to provide opportunities to eat a wide variety of foods.

Taking a doggie bag after a meal out—for example, half a sandwich that wasn't touched—and then finding a local shelter or a homeless person to feed provides priceless opportunities for character development.

Most important, you can use this period to teach your child the principles of good nutrition. You won't necessarily see the rewards now, but you will see them later. This is a good opportunity to get a food chart or a play kitchen and start exploring the food pyramid. Help your child learn which foods go into which food category. Cut out pictures of foods from magazines and make your own food pyramid. Point our where these foods come from. Visit a farm and see how carrots grow. You can make a nutritional impact on your preschooler that will last a lifetime, including fostering interest in new foods.

> FYI: The typical three-year-old needs about 44 calories per pound of body weight per day, but by age four, children need only about 40 calories per pound of body weight per day. The expected monthly weight gain will also drop.

Dietary Needs of Preschoolers

Preschoolers usually eat on a schedule similar to the traditional school-age child. They get up early in the morning, hungry, and eat breakfast. They have a significant outpouring of energy in school and need a hearty mid-morning snack. They stop for lunch, then have another period of play, and go home to a healthful snack. Then it's a few hours of quiet play or even a nap followed by a light dinner, bath, and bed.

- *Increase the offerings of calcium-rich foods.* Your child needs about 16 to 24 ounces of milk or calcium-rich food, somewhat more than he did as a toddler.
- *Add more protein.* The preschooler's diet requires more protein than it did during the toddler years.

Kids in the Kitchen

Three-year-olds can

- wrap potatoes in foil for baking
- shake liquids in covered container
- knead and shape yeast dough
- spread soft spreads
- pour liquids
- place things in trash
- mix ingredients

Four-year-olds can

- peel oranges or hard-cooked eggs
- mash bananas using a fork
- set the table
- cut parsley or green onions with dull scissors

- *Add more fiber.* The preschooler needs more fiber than before. Salads are really helpful here. Children aren't big bran eaters at any age, but fruits and vegetables are good choices for preschoolers as part of their meals. Try including different dried fruits in the lunch box.
- *Add calories.* The preschooler's diet has to be higher in calories than the toddler's. That means more starch and protein, not more sugar. When your four-year-old reaches out for an energy snack, half a peanut-butter sandwich is in order!

- *Set regular mealtimes.* Their lifestyle doesn't allow for such frequent snacking, so the traditional "three meals a day plus a snack or two" now makes some sense for preschoolers.
- *Provide snacks with long-lasting energy.* The best snack for a four-year-old is something that will fuel him longer, such as cheese and crackers. This is also the age when children take food along with them, so your snacks have to make sense for carrying along. They can't be gooey and soft because they're not going to make it through half a day of school. Preschoolers need food that will give them lasting energy; more complex foods such as nuts (watch out for allergic reactions), seeds, and beans—in the so-called trail-mix combinations—are good choices. You and your child can mix your own, adding the items she particularly likes. You still need to be vigilant, though less so, regarding food size and risk of choking.
- *Supervise snacking.* Be sure your child is not running with food in his hand or mouth. At school, children should be seated and supervised at snack time.
- *Make veggies fun when possible.* Vegetables are important, but be creative. For example, carrot sticks are perfect dippers for anything from puréed fruits to yogurt or cheese dips.

Now you can finally stop stocking a variety of milks in your refrigerator. The entire family can drink low-fat or nonfat milk if you want to.

Turn healthful foods into fun foods

Dear Dr. Paula,

From the time Todd was three, we started making evening snacks out of healthful foods made in the shape of things he was excited about, like a rocket ship. Most nights he eats a standing banana surrounded by a "jet stream" of sliced apple "fuel" with dabs of peanut butter in the trail of fire.

Todd's mom

Dear Todd's mom,

That's very creative, and I will pass that on to parents. Here's another creative idea shared by another mom. Her motto is, "If you cut it, they will eat it." Janet's mom says that Janet may not pick up an apple and bite into it, but she will eat it if it is cut into slices. She even uses a muffin tin to entice her preschooler to eat. In each muffin hole she puts different stacks of healthy foods. She adds pretty cupcake paper, which makes it even more appealing.

Preschoolers and breakfast

Breakfast really *is* the most important meal of the day. After all, your child just fasted for eight hours or more. That's why it is called "break fast." Your child should face the day like a lion, not like a lump. If your child is expected to go to preschool at 8:00 A.M. and learn new things, all the more reason to eat breakfast.

Most American children don't eat breakfast. You must sit down with your child and take the extra five minutes to eat breakfast yourself, even if it's only "Kellogg's in the morning" or a breakfast bar. I don't expect many parents to present their child with a stack of pancakes freshly made from flour and buckwheat, but I do expect a single serving of ready-to-eat cereal. Or just rip open a packet of instant oatmeal and add warm water. Throw in a slice of apple or orange and you get the good-parent award!

Preschoolers and lunch

It's time to help them pick out a cute little lunch box and what goes in it. You still want to be very cautious (don't send peanuts or popcorn), but you can be more explorative in your selections. Safety while eating remains an issue.

The preschooler who was a finicky toddler is more likely to try foods that other children are eating when they are sitting together at the same table at school. Keep these thoughts in mind: If you're sending snacks, be a little more creative and do not be too concerned that your child won't eat any of it. The chances are good that even if your child doesn't like what's in his own lunch box, he will trade with someone else for something he does like.

The other thing to remember is that you have an important opportunity to influence the quality of the snack and lunch program in your child's school, and it begins with the preschool programs—speak up and become involved. Salad bars introduced in preschool result in children who eat more salad. From preschool

Salad bars introduced in preschool result in children who eat more salad.

through kindergarten or first grade, some schools offer a supervised salad bar; the child selects and the teacher puts the food into his bowl. This opportunity also lends itself to teaching children about what's healthy, what kinds of choices there are, and what constitutes a portion. If your school doesn't have a salad bar, it won't take much influence from parents to get one. Be willing to offer to help in the time-consuming process of serving so that it goes smoothly.

Rules for dinner

Preschool children like rules. This is the perfect age to make rules about how you come to the table. Announce matter-of-factly: "Dinner's ready; everybody wash up." Make it a habit and teach by example. Elbows off the table, napkin on the lap, don't talk with your mouth full. If you keep modeling, it becomes second nature. We have rules in my house: No phone calls during dinner, no sitting in front of the television, and no reading material brought to the table.

Eating In

Today's families rarely eat a meal together on a regular basis. Not so long ago, it was popular to have dinner on a table in front of the television—"TV dinners," as they were called. Dinnertime should be a regular family event for your preschooler, as opposed to your toddler, who ate only when he needed to. The preschooler is part of the table scene, but don't expect meals to last too long.

Kids can be expected to enjoy and learn things at meals. A preschooler is not the challenge a toddler was with regard to mealtime. You won't have to remove play dough from the mouth of your four-year-old. Somewhere between the ages of three and five you have opportunities to work with your preschooler on skills that will grow from child skills into adult skills over time.

Manners

It's finally the time to bring out the "Miss Manners" manual you've been saving. Manners do count now, but it requires patience and good humor to establish them as a regular part of mealtime. Manners are not something we come to naturally, but we like to see them in others.

We are mostly not happy with caveman-style eating. Most cultures use implements to eat with. Forks and spoons and eventually knives are useful tools. Of course, setting an example all along is important. But at this age, you can teach a child the correct way to hold a fork and praise him when he does it right. You can even give your preschool child a dull butter knife and teach him how to use it for cutting food instead of playing war with it at the table. You are helping him to become confident and competent and to improve his fine-motor abilities—all while teaching important social skills.

A common mistake a lot of parents make is to continue to cut their child's food. Your child can begin to learn to do this for himself. Start by letting your child cut up pancakes. This exercise is about learning new skills, so be sure to be enthusiastic and supportive of your child's efforts. If you don't start when your child is young, it is hard to retrench and teach the skills later.

You may soon consider having friends over for dinner, and you can expect less than a debacle with children at the table. All those things are not only possible, but it is your obligation now to begin to expect it. However, you have to teach it before you can expect it. Just remember that "practice makes perfect" in time.

Eating Out

Fast food

Fast food is not always bad. There are even occasions when it can be a fun family event. In some ways, it is today's version of a picnic. We don't have many places to picnic in the city, so we go to McDonald's and spread out our napkins and eat with the family.

Choose carefully. Someone who's ordered the double cheeseburger with fries is not choosing as well as the child who orders a single burger with lettuce and tomato and an ear of corn or baked potato. Or how about having your kids try the McVeggie burger? You can even order salads at Burger King these days.

> Make sure you don't eat fast food too fast or too often.

Restaurants

It's time to go back to the diner or coffee shop as a family. A general rule of thumb: If your child is ready to walk in without a stroller, he is ready to go to a restaurant. From the age of four, my daughter loved to have a special meal out with me at a

"restaurant with napkins."
It wasn't very often, because, in fact, she wasn't very good at it and inevitably something would spill on the tablecloth. But we kept at it and it got better each time. Sometimes aim for "special" because food is more

A general rule of thumb: If a child is ready to walk in without a stroller, he is ready to go to a restaurant.

than just for nutrition. Food, after all, is an important entrée to relationships. We negotiate, have dates, socialize, and cooperate over food.

Be aware that kids aren't always in the mood to be brave when it comes to new foods. Let your preschooler order what she will eat, and don't expect exotic choices—the new environment and the "lucky" waiter are exotic enough for most four-year-olds.

Tip: Have a "dinner out" at home for your three-to-four-year-old. Put a napkin over your arm, and make believe you are the waiter, or let your child be the waiter. Let him serve. Make believe that you are dining in a foreign restaurant. Keep pretending to try new foods—it is less threatening this way.

> Dear Dr. Paula,
>
> We went out to lunch after church, and it was one of the best restaurant outings we have had with three little ones so far. We have found that Mexican restaurants seem to be best because the atmosphere is loud, there are chips immediately available, and the older girls love warm tortillas with butter. They always order quesadillas and rice and eat pretty decently.
>
> Mom of three girls

Dear "little girls" mom,

*Olé! You have struck gold with your dining choice.
For some families, it's Chinese food. Of course,
outings like this don't happen every day. But enjoy
them when they do. It makes for great memories.*

Choose restaurants carefully

You can easily figure out if a restaurant is "child friendly." That
means paper tablecloths, or place mats, crayons on the table,
and a child's menu. Find out what is on the menu before going,
and make sure there is something for your child to eat. When
you get there, be very nice to the waiter. Let him know you
would like the child's main course to come out at the same time
as your appetizer, because three-year-olds are not patient. Let
the waiter know in advance that you won't be having dessert so
he will not come over and say, "Dessert, anyone?" Ask for the
check when entrées are delivered.

Outside Influences

This is the age when children are influenced by friends, teachers,
television, everything around them. You are less in control of
your child's food than ever before. For the first time, your child
will regularly be eating without you, often in a room with other
children.

In fact, most children eat better at school than they do at
home, and that has to do more with the environment in school
than anything else. It's not the great school lunches. It's partly
peer pressure. Your child is probably hungry after he's been
playing for hours. And they're all sitting together mimicking one
another without a parent putting pressure on them to eat.

Lunch in school is where all the socialization takes place. It's usually where the kids figure out who their friends are, where they sit, who they sit next to. Often preschoolers are allowed to trade food. It is an activity that's fun, and it encourages sharing. There are healthy snacks that you can send that your child won't be ashamed to share. This is very important; a bag of salty pretzels is a lot more healthful than a bag of potato chips, yet it's still trade-worthy. If you send your child with saltless pretzels, he may not accomplish a trade. Applesauce is also a "yes," but pudding is more likely to get successfully bartered. (And there are more healthful chocolate puddings to select from. Your child won't taste the difference.) Also in your child's lunch box can go things such as little toys. Your child can even trade stickers or pencils. Don't limit yourself. You and your child can pack his lunch box together for the next day.

At the end of the day, when you open up the lunch box, use that time to talk about school. If your child's lunch box is full when he gets home, don't assume he is not eating. Ask the teacher what's going on. Chances are good that he ate someone else's lunch.

If your child has food allergies, the conditions for bartering have to be very strictly controlled. That includes not only warning your child's teachers but, in the case of peanuts, separating your child from the other kids during mealtime. Trading food with other children can be hazardous. Some schools have actually outlawed peanuts altogether to avoid the risks.

8

Preschooler Roadblocks

Dear Dr. Paula,

Sam is four and a half and still eats the same three foods he started with when he was two. He will eat crackers, sometimes with jelly on them, scrambled eggs, and bananas. At preschool, the other kids make fun of him because his snack box is "weird." I only pack banana slices and Wheat Thins because I can't pack a scrambled egg and he won't touch the hard-boiled kind I tried to send. I'm worried about his nutrition, but also about his strange food choices. What can I do to get him to try new foods?

Desperate mom

Dear Desperate mom,

Sam's food pickiness is a leftover from the toddler years, and he does need to move on despite his reluctance to do so. First, broaden his food choices in his snack box even if you are right and he is not likely to touch any of it. At least his school friends may be willing to trade with him. Sam might even show interest in something in another child's box, but he won't have access to it unless his lunch box is appealing to the other children as well.

Don't worry too much about balanced nutrition at school. You can work with him at home to achieve some balance, and I would begin that mission with the use of the Children's Food Pyramid, available from the USDA. The chart is colorful and child friendly, and you can ask Sam to help cut out pictures from magazines that fit onto the chart in the different categories. Take advantage of his expanding curiosity. He is at the age when new projects like this might appeal to him. You might even involve the teacher with a project that involves nutrition facts. Good luck!

The Preschool Picky Eater

The preschool picky eater was most likely a toddler whose parents allowed or encouraged him to be a picky eater. Maybe as a toddler he ate only three foods—rice, pasta, and yogurt—and his parents never even put out other foods. They figured, "What's the point? He won't eat it anyway." Those parents took what was an age- and stage-appropriate food pickiness and grew it into a more lasting behavioral problem. Every time the child ate rice, pasta, and yogurt, mom and dad were satisfied, but other foods should have been offered regularly also. Then the child might have decided, "Maybe I should try those foods. Mommy eats those and so does daddy." That's how you avoid creating the preschool-aged picky eater.

A preschooler is a child who thinks more about things and can control his parents by what and how he eats. This can take the form of the child who gets ridiculously picky about how the food should be presented. "I want it shaped in a star, and if it touches the string beans I won't eat it at all." If this is reinforced by parents who comply to all of his demands, it can lead to an assortment of food disorders.

If you don't nip this pickiness early, you'll end up with a child who controls *you* with food. The parent of a toddler who says, "Oh, please eat this and I'll give you a Pokémon" leads to a preschool child who says, "I'll eat this if I get a new Pokémon."

A child's cognitive growth in the preschool years enables him to comprehend what it means when you say, "I know you prefer that to be in the shape of a dinosaur, but you can eat it anyway. Otherwise you will be hungry later." Do this simply and with little emotion. Practice and you will get better and better. In time your child will understand and at least pick at something. Don't pull food away like the mean stepmothers in scary tales and say, "Then go to bed without your supper!" Rather, let the food sit out for a while. *You are trying to reeducate a child who has learned from you how to control you with food.* When you are "fixing" a problem, you can expect regression, and the first stop in this case will be back to toddlerhood. Expect some tantrums, but stick to your guns.

> Dear Dr. Paula,
>
> Abby, age four, awoke grumpy and on edge. She demanded a pink cup to drink out of when handed the blue one. I should have said, "This is it, kiddo, deal with it. This time the cup is blue." But instead I poured the juice into a pink cup and kept peace for a little while longer. Did I win the battle, but lose the war?
>
> Abby's dad

Dear Abby's dad,

It's time for a truce. Preschool-aged children like Abby easily regress to toddler behaviors when they are tired. Rather than reinforce the setback, you could appeal to the "big girl" growing up inside her and sit quietly nearby. Touch her hand if she's not too irritable and say, "Rough day? Sometimes I have days when I can't seem to get the pink-cup thing right. Maybe later you'll feel better." Then move the scene out of the kitchen, bringing along the blue cup in case she remembers she's thirsty. Put the focus on the emotion, not the obsession.

Solutions for the picky eater

Don't ridicule or deny the child's feelings. Cooperate to a reasonable extent in order to teach.

Don't cater to the pickiness of a preschooler. There's nothing wrong with offering him the plate with compartments (for the kid who doesn't like his foods to touch), but don't bring it with you on play dates or to restaurants. It's no longer age- or stage-appropriate to lug it along.

Avoid treating a preschooler like a toddler. Take advantage of your child's growing ability to reason. When your preschooler has a hissy fit because you didn't cut the sandwich in the "right" shape, explain what his choices are but don't try to recut the sandwich to his specifications. That would be encouraging your child to be inflexible. I've seen ten-year-olds practically beat up their parents in restaurants if the food isn't brought out exactly as they want it. You can imagine the adult version of this.

Let the child help you prepare foods when possible. This gives her some input about what she eats. This is a good way for preschoolers to develop skills such as fine-motor coordination, independence, and decisionmaking.

Set an example. You may set examples by eating foods that are in the form that your preschooler is rejecting and even say, "Gee, I like it sometimes when my food is square-shaped instead of a circle or dipped in sauce."

The picky eater at school

This is the child who doesn't join the others when everybody is eating snacks, causing the teachers not to be happy with that child. The picky eater is not a popular child in school. He is an annoyance to the teacher and to the other kids. Others will ridicule and embarrass him. If, however, your picky-eating preschooler isn't as picky at school, it might be related to the positive impact of peer pressure at school.

> Picky eating affects more than just nutrition.

Return of the Dessert Monster

Coupling dessert with *any* behavior is a mistake. Dessert should not be used as a reward or withheld as punishment. Sometimes it is at the root of temper tantrums, moody behavior, rage at parents, and even food disorders. "If you don't eat your peas, you don't get dessert." Or, "If you are good, mommy has a special dessert for you." It all amounts to using food to control.

If you made the mistake of teaching your toddler to live for dessert, you can still correct this. I know a very clever mom who puts the dessert out at the same time as the rest of the meal, and her child knows that she can eat as much as she wants of it. More often than not, she will only eat a little bit since the tension attached to it has been removed. If you have the dessert monster on your hands, I strongly suggest that you take the emphasis off dessert.

The (Early) Dinner Hour?

> Dear Dr. Paula,
>
> I always try to have the family eat together. But after preschool, Timmy is so hungry he could eat a horse. I can't hold him until dinnertime, so I wind up feeding him early. Then I just hate it when he's sitting alone in front of the TV while his older brother and baby sister are joining me and daddy for dinner.
>
> Timmy's mom

> *Dear Timmy's mom,*
>
> *You're right. Don't exclude your child from the family meal just because he's on a different nutritional time frame. Find ways to include Timmy in family mealtime, perhaps by offering him a small snack while the rest of the family eats the main meal.*

Often we don't have dinner ready for our preschoolers at the "right" hour. They may be hungry earlier, and in an effort to have dinner as a family, we give a snack at 4:00 P.M. Then your child really isn't hungry when the family sits down to dinner. You have to figure out a way to manage this. Don't assume that you can give him a rich snack and he will have an appetite and interest in food later. Offer a small version of dinner at 4:00 P.M. That's more nutritionally appropriate to the needs of his body.

Then later, when the family gathers, offer a smaller plate with a dip and a couple of carrot sticks so he can be included in the meal.

Outside Influences, Again

At this age some children may come home and announce, "Jason's mommy lets Jason eat Twinkies." Now is the time for you to start practicing saying, "Jason's family does things one way, and our family does things another way." You may feel bad about this, and your child may not like you very much for the moment, but he will get used to it. You are setting a standard for all time. When your child is eight or even eighteen, and he wants to do something you wouldn't approve of, you will still say, "That's Jason's family . . ." And you won't have to finish the thought. Start now and you are in great shape. Delay and you will have big problems. Besides, when your child says, "Jason's mom lets him eat Twinkies for dinner," he is probably exaggerating or repeating Jason's fantasy meal. If it is true, Jason may be destined for obesity. Don't denigrate the other family, just make it clear what your family's rules are and that they are supreme.

Before play dates, you might want to speak to the other parent and set up rules. There will be less reason for disappointment when your child comes home. ("I ate Cracker Jacks all day long at Jimmy's house. Why can't I eat them here?") Bear in mind that not all parents are willing to modify rules just because you asked them to. In some cases, you may discover you don't want your child playing at Jimmy's house at all. *If you disagree totally about food choices, that probably is a home where you would disagree about many other issues as well.*

On the other hand, you can be a good influence and strengthen another family by having a dialogue about how your kid "gets crazed when he eats too many cookies, so would you mind if I send along some snacks that I prefer he eat?" That mother may be curious to see what you send, and her child may try that food because it is a novelty.

> Dear Dr. Paula,
>
> My son had a play date with John, and John's mother called and said, "When my son comes over, would you mind if I send along a bottle of Sprite?" She knew that I don't let my son drink soda. At first I said, "OK." And then I thought, wait a minute. What kind of special food need is soda? John couldn't spend one afternoon without it? The more I thought about it, the more annoyed I got. So I called her back and said, "I was thinking about your request, and it would be really difficult for me to explain to my child why your child has soda. In our house, we don't drink soda. Can your son drink water, juice, or milk instead?" John's mom argued her son's right to drink soda, so we just called off the play date.
>
> Frank's mom

> *Dear Frank's mom,*
>
> *Good decision!*

Holiday Horrors

> Dear Dr. Paula,
>
> This year my kids found Halloween horrible because no matter how much or what type of candy they got,

there was no way we could come to some peaceful arrangement about consuming it. Now I'm even dreading Thanksgiving and Christmas.

Help!

Candy lovers' mom

Dear Candy lovers' mom,

You are not alone. Holidays make everyone nutritionally nervous. We tend to overeat at holidays, and there is less opportunity to put our rules into place once the holiday comes. There are usually too many people around. The entire event can be ruined by your child's food-related behavior. Unless you plan in advance and have structure in place, you are heading for bad memories. (What's the opposite of a Kodak moment?) Halloween especially requires negotiation before the candy is hoarded. Try agreeing on the number of candies your child can expect to consume during the evening and over the next few days.

General tips for holiday celebrations include the following:

- Never arrive hungry.
- Bring snacks that you feel comfortable letting your preschooler choose.
- Relax some of your usual rules, especially if you are in someone else's home; for example, dessert may take center stage occasionally at Grandma's.
- Let your child know what kind of arrangements to expect. This may be your child's first experience at a buffet or his first meal sitting with his cousins.

Television and Food

By this age, you will find your children are mesmerized by television programs and commercials. That is quite intentional on the part of the advertisers. The food commercials are more magical than anything else, because they are aimed literally for the gut. Children fly through the air with junk food in their hands. There is often a special toy inside the box, something you have to send away for. There's no money to be made advertising green veggies to kids. Ah, if we could only package broccoli with a toy!

Television is absolutely guilty of the crime of fostering bad food habits. Your child is eager to have what that kid or adorable animal is jumping up for in the commercial. The food dances, the food has smiley faces, saying "Buy me!" It is incredibly seductive, and it affects all ages. To this day, I can't walk through the aisles of the supermarket without my teenagers asking for a specific brand of cereal that they have never eaten, because they saw the product on television.

> Point out how foods look different in the ads than they do in real life. For example, buy a McDonald's hamburger just for the purpose of opening it up and comparing it to the TV ad. Does it really look as good "in person" as it does on TV? Teach your children how to be media savvy.

Preschoolers and Obesity

Be aware that this is the age where obesity can take root. (See Chapter 13. As a toddler, your child was racing around, and now he is less active. Suddenly some preschoolers seem to be getting fat. They are now dividing up at preschool by who can dodge the ball and who can't. Even at this young age, children get separated by their prowess and talents. They discover their physical capabilities and limitations, and others categorize them by these realities. The child who is a couch potato at home is likely to just sit there on the sports field at school as well. There are huge emotional consequences in this as well as medical ones.

9

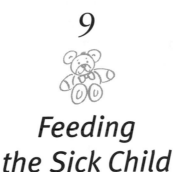

Feeding the Sick Child

Dear Dr. Paula,

My four-year-old son, Jack, has been sick for a week. His cold seems to be improving but he hasn't had a decent meal in days. I can never remember whether it's "feed a cold and starve a fever" or the opposite. Whatever it is, Jack just isn't eating. What should I do? I'm really worried about him.

Jack's mom

Dear Jack's mom,

I never got the point of that old adage either, but Jack may just be recovering slowly. Sick kids just don't eat much, but make sure he is getting plenty of liquids.

The Basics

Here are a few facts that will help both you and your sick child. Parents can't help feeling vulnerable when their child doesn't feel

well. It's comforting to know how and what to feed your child
to help hasten his recovery or at least to not make things worse.

Always have a stash of bland foods and rehydration solution,
such as Pedialyte, on hand to help banish the blahs. Bland foods
include applesauce, eggs, potato, banana, rice, crackers, and
pasta.

When a child is sick, she is usually not hungry. Therefore she
won't eat as much as she normally would. In the case of a sick
toddler, her intake may be next to nothing, because toddlers eat
very little even when they feel fine.

*Anyone who is sick needs liquids more than they need regular
food.* And you need even *more fluids than usual* to replace what
you are losing when you are sick. If your child has a stomach
virus, he is losing fluids in the form of diarrhea and by throwing
up. If your child has only a fever, he still loses fluid through his
skin by evaporation—that's how the body cools itself. If he has
a headache or sore throat, he loses fluid because he breathes
more rapidly. When you breathe, you also exhale water vapor,
and this extra loss needs to be replaced. Almost any illness
results in a net loss of fluid. Couple that with not feeling like
eating, and your child can easily get dehydrated. You need more
fluids when you are sick. (See the box on page 121, "Signs of
Dehydration.")

*Don't give your sick child any food or liquids you wouldn't
ordinarily give.* Don't create bad food habits just because your
child is sick. If soda is forbidden in your house, don't rush out
to get ginger ale because you heard it's good for an upset
stomach. There are better solutions, such as chamomile tea.
Most childhood illnesses are not so serious that you need to
discard all your rules. I've known parents who are so concerned
that a slightly dehydrated child needs salt that they give him
potato chips. (Soon they will have a well child who wants

Signs of Dehydration

- sunken soft spot (for infants)
- weak-sounding cry
- dry mouth, lips, and tongue
- cries without tears
- doesn't urinate for hours
- listless or irritable behavior
- sudden increase in temper tantrums

chips.) There are a lot of better ways to replace salt that are nutritionally balanced. Electrolyte solutions are best for this, but clear broths and saltines also work well.

FYI: You Might Not Know . . .

Milk does not create mucus. No matter what you have heard, this is not supported by scientific fact. In one recent study, army recruits were infected with a respiratory virus. Half of the sick group was allowed milk products, and half had no dairy products at all. Then they measured mucus production. There was no difference. However, you may be advised to cut back on dairy products when an illness involves vomiting or diarrhea. In the case of diarrhea, you want to avoid foods that are hard on the gut, because your gut is already "busy" having diarrhea. Eating dairy products results in gassiness and cramps.

Feed the flu. Some parents have been told that when a child has diarrhea, they should stop giving the child all food. Most recent research has shown that, on the contrary, your child will recover more quickly if given small amounts of carefully chosen bland food throughout the illness. New rule: Introduce normal foods in small amounts as early as possible during stomach flu. Avoid sugary foods, because sugar quickens the movement of the gut, which only adds to the problem when a child has diarrhea.

Bland foods include applesauce, eggs, potato, banana, rice, crackers, and pasta.

A vomiting child still needs water. Don't keep fluids away from a child because she is vomiting. She needs fluids even if every time you give some, she throws up. The key is in the timing: Give only sips, but offer sips every few minutes and gradually build in quantity as the vomiting becomes less frequent. A quick rinse and spit with plain water after vomiting will also help prevent dental decay and clear the "yucky" taste.

Common Questions Concerning Sick Infants

My five-month-old has a really stuffy nose. She can't suck the bottle or my breast. What do I do?
Infant nutrition is particularly important when your child is sick because she loses fluids quickly. Dehydration can make a child really sick—more so than the illness itself. First of all, baby must have clear airways in order to suck to get fluid and nutrition. This is especially vital before the age of six months, when all she can take is liquids.

Clear her nose: Put saline nose drops into the baby's nostrils. Turn the shower on hot and steam up the bathroom. Then feed her while sitting in the steamy room or directly afterward. The mucus will begin to thin, making it easier to feed. Also offer your stuffy baby sips of plain water between feedings to replace fluid losses.

My eight-month-old baby has diarrhea. Everything I give her seems to come out the other end. She's not vomiting. What do I feed her?
A baby who has diarrhea without vomiting needs a gut rest. (Make sure you consult with your pediatrician.) But she doesn't need to be starved, or you'll wind up with a dehydrated baby. If you are breast-feeding, continue to breast-feed. If you are formula-feeding, you might be advised to give an electrolyte solution or soy formula instead. Foods that are good for your baby include starchy foods such as cereal, bread, bananas, and potato. Avoid prunes, plums, peaches, and other fruits that make the child "go."

Should I give rice to my child with diarrhea? I heard that rice constipates.
Processed white rice can constipate, but whole-grain brown rice can actually loosen stools. Brown rice is rich in fiber. Here's a little-known tip: When you boil any rice, you may use the starchy water to mix with banana or applesauce to increase the binding power of those foods.

My child has vomiting *and* diarrhea. What do I feed him?
This is tricky, because of the vomiting. The more fluid that is leaving the body, the faster the child can become dehydrated. Start with rehydration solutions, such as Pedialyte. Once the vomiting slows, add small bits of starchy foods. If you withhold food, you could prolong the illness. Therefore, within forty-eight hours, regardless if there is still some diarrhea or vomiting, slowly add back some food. Avoid dairy products.

Common Questions Concerning Sick Toddlers

My two-year-old has had a horrible cold for a week. She barely eats anything. The doctor says she's getting dehydrated.

Don't forget that toddlers are famous for being obstinate. The sick toddler needs to be cajoled. They also need you to help clear their nose. They are usually cranky and irritable. Just like an infant, they can get dehydrated, and they need fluids. One of my favorite ways to get a sick toddler to eat is to put the child in the bathtub and float the food to them. Watermelon is a great source of water and sugar, and it floats. Just cut it into small triangles and launch. You may be thinking: How unhygienic! If you can't tolerate the idea, just put some on a tray on the side of the tub and invite your toddler to a bath party. Somehow being in the bath helps the appetite appear. Or arrange a picnic on the floor. You want to give toddlers food that does the job quickly and is appealing. Try using a cookie cutter to make fun shapes of cheese on crackers.

Should I give my child vitamin C so he won't get a cold in the first place?

There's no proof that taking vitamin C prevents colds. There is some evidence, however, that high-dose vitamin C can shorten the length of respiratory viruses by a day or two. That's a good thing. (Children shouldn't be given more than 500 milligrams a day.)

My child has the blahs. He's had a sore throat for days. What should I feed him?

Comfort foods are good—the same foods we would crave, like mashed potatoes, which slide right down. And it's OK to add butter. Children will almost always eat pudding. Sometimes ice cream and fruit ices work best, because the cold numbs the pain and children like them.

My sick toddler won't eat much. She's not dehydrated because she's drinking plenty of fluids, but I would like to get some "real" food into her.
Any child who is sick won't eat much. Don't think in terms of balanced nutrition or the food pyramid when your child is sick. The goal is to make sure the child gets fluids and small amounts of bland foods. If your child has a sore throat, offer cold liquids. If your child has a headache, then avoid cold foods.

Common Questions Concerning Sick Preschoolers

My five-year-old has been sick for five days. She is just starting to feel a little better. She's been watching television. Would it be so terrible this one time if I let her eat in front of the TV?
Being sick can get very boring. A little chicken soup and crackers in front of the TV won't hurt. The only problem is that when she gets well, she will want the same privilege. Be prepared to reestablish your rules.

My child gets ear infections all the time. Every time we finish the antibiotic she gets thrush or a vaginal itch and discharge. I dread it—what can we do?
When your sick child is on antibiotics, try to give her plain real yogurt. Yogurt contains acidophilus, which helps to restore the balance of intestinal "flora," a vital step in recovery from antibiotic-induced diarrhea. Unlike other dairy products, yogurt does not irritate the gut.

My son has chicken pox. He's not really sick, but he's very cranky and itchy. He won't eat much. What can I do?

A kid with chicken pox would do well to sit in an oatmeal bath—for the itching, not for the eating. If his throat hurts, he needs cold things like sherbet and fruit ices and appropriate pain relief (ask his pediatrician). After the first few days, he will feel better and his appetite will return. Try peanut butter for a child recovering from chicken pox. Peanut butter is high in protein, and it can be played with—your child can put it on a cracker and make a face in it or dip into it with an apple. It's even OK if he sucks it off his fingers.

My preschooler is a mess. She has a stomach bug with both diarrhea and vomiting. What can I do for her?

Make sure she doesn't get dehydrated. Give small, frequent quantities of well-balanced fluids—preferably rehydration solution. Unfortunately, older children are often unwilling to drink those solutions. Take a rehydration solution and add to it a little bit of a fluid they love—like a fruit drink—to make it more acceptable. A child who is losing fluids needs more than just plain water.

The standard diet for children with diarrhea is BRATTS: *Bananas, Rice, Apples, Toast, Tea,* and *Soup.* Some fatty foods should be on the list too, such as peanut butter and scrambled eggs. The net balance of food going in should be more than whatever is coming out.

Remember that your sick child will turn back into your well child soon enough. So always make sure she has plenty of fluids and appropriate food, and don't forget to add lots of "TLC" to the menu.

PART TWO

Food Facts and Fictions

10

The Food Pyramid Explained

*I*n 1992, the United States Department of Agriculture (USDA) Center for Nutrition Policy and Promotion released a new guide to children's nutrition. Based on the already existing Adult Food Guide Pyramid, the New Food Guide Pyramid for Young Children was created as a resource for parents for feeding children ages two through six. It is based on extensive research about the eating patterns of American children and includes foods children actually eat.

The key message of the children's food guide is variety. Children should be encouraged to eat a wide variety of foods so that they will obtain all the nutrients necessary for sound health.

The Children's Food Guide Pyramid also depicts children exercising as a reminder that good nutrition includes regular daily physical activity. Probably the best aspect of the pyramid is the educational opportunities it provides for parents and teachers. The pictures are child-friendly and colorful.

- Important adaptations need to be made when using the pyramid for two-to-three-year-old toddlers as compared to four-to-six-year-olds. Parents need to know that the younger age group needs fewer calories and therefore requires smaller servings.
- Another unwritten but vital message in the food guide is that fat intake needs to decrease over the two-to-six-year-old age period so that by age five, children are receiving no more than 30 percent of their total daily calories from fat, much like the current adult recommendations.

How Many Calories per Day?

Age	Weight Gain Expected Monthly	Total Daily Calories Needed	Calories Needed per Pound, per Day
0–3 mos.	2 lbs.	400–500	52
3–6 mos.	1 1/4 lbs.	500–550	50
6–9 mos.	1 lb.	550–600	44
9–12 mos.	3/4 lb.	600–800	44
1–3 years	1/2 lb.	800–1,200	44
4–6 years	1/4 lb.	1,200–2,000	40–44

Examples:
- A typical eight-month-old weighing 15 pounds needs about 660 calories a day.
- A typical eighteen-month-old weighing 23 pounds needs about 1,000 calories a day but will gain very little weight each month compared with the eight-month-old.
- A typical four-year-old weighing 40 pounds needs approximately 1,600 calories a day and will gain even more slowly than the toddler.

The Children's Food Guide Pyramid

It is recommended that you offer a variety of foods from the five major food groups each day and that you let your children decide which ones and how much of each to eat. A reproduction of this food guide pyramid appears on page 132.

- At the base of the pyramid is the *grain group*. Most of a child's food comes from this group. Grains are important for providing vitamins, minerals, complex carbohydrates, and fiber.
- The next level includes *fruits and vegetables,* which also provide vitamins, minerals, and fiber and are good for quick energy. Your child needs fewer of these than of the grains.
- Moving up the pyramid, the next category is the *milk group*. The foods in this category are vital for providing calcium for a growing child.
- The *meat group* includes many protein sources, including some foods that are technically not "meat." For example, in this category we find eggs, beans, peas, and peanut butter. This group also includes poultry and fish. All of these foods are important for providing protein, iron, and zinc in the diet.
- At the top of the pyramid is a small area intended to depict foods that contain mostly *fat and sugar.* Although our children need some of these substances, foods in the tip contain many calories but *few* vitamins and minerals. Your children should eat fewer foods from this category than any other.

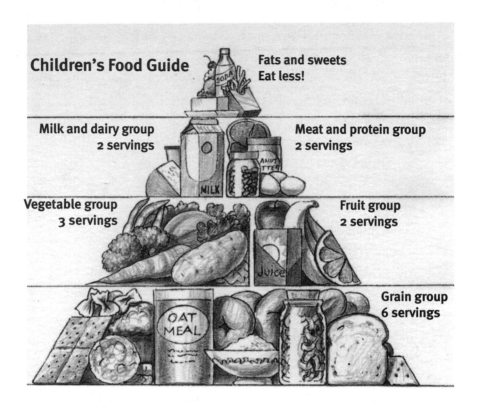

Children's Food Guide Pyramid

Child-Friendly Food Choices

Below is a summary of child-friendly food choices and serving sizes. Children aged two to three are separated from the four- and five-year-olds in this plan mainly by serving size. Keep in mind that toddler choices will be more limited because toddlers tend to be choosier about what they eat.

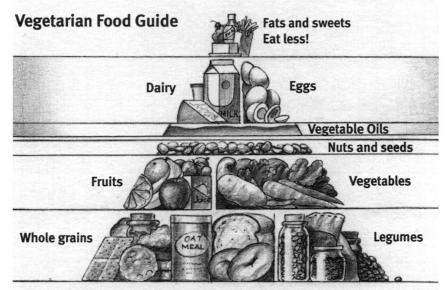

Vegetarian Food Guide

Fats and sweets
Eat less!

Dairy

Eggs

Vegetable Oils

Nuts and seeds

Fruits

Vegetables

Whole grains

Legumes

Traditional Vegetarian Diet Pyramid

Grain group

Choose six servings each day from the following list. (The pyramid recommends that at least three of the six choices be of a whole- or mixed-grain type, rather than processed or "white.")

Toddler (ages 1 1/2–3)
   2 tablespoons of cooked brown rice
   2 tablespoons of cooked oatmeal
   1/2 ounce ready-to-eat cereal
   1/2 slice bread
   1/4 bagel
   3 small crackers
   1/2 small pancake
   1/4 cup cooked grits

4 animal crackers (any animals)

1/2 small muffin or biscuit

Preschooler (ages 4–5)

1/2 cup cooked brown rice

2 graham cracker squares

1/2 cup oatmeal

3 cups popcorn

3 rice cakes

1 slice bread

2 taco shells

1/2 cup spaghetti

1 small roll

1/2 hamburger bun or hot dog bun

1 ounce cereal

1 small muffin

4 small cookies

Vegetable group

Choose two to three servings a day.

Toddler

1 cooked broccoli spear

5 french fries

2 tablespoons peas

1/2 cup bean soup

2 slices of cucumber

2 tablespoons of spaghetti sauce or ketchup

3 cherry tomatoes

Preschooler
  1 cup lettuce
  2 broccoli spears
  7 short carrot sticks
  1 medium ear corn
  1 medium baked potato
  1 medium plantain
  1/2 cup beans (black, kidney, pinto, garbanzo, or black-eyed)
  1/2 cup cooked green beans
  1/2 cup coleslaw
  1 cup vegetable soup
  1 medium tomato

Fruit group

Choose two servings per day.

Toddler
  1 very small melon wedge
  1/2 orange
  3 strawberries
  1/4 cup watermelon
  1 small apricot
  1 slice dried apricot
  4 tablespoons applesauce
  6 grapes
  1/4 cup fruit cocktail
  1/2 banana

Preschooler
  1/2 cup blueberries
  3/4 cup 100 percent orange juice
  1/2 grapefruit
  1 orange
  6 strawberries
  1 banana
  2 canned pineapple slices
  1/2 medium mango
  1/4 medium papaya
  1 kiwi
Note: The pyramid depicts a juice box as a serving in the fruit category. The recommended serving size is three-fourths of a juice box, or 4 ounces. However, be careful not to offer juice as the main fruit choice, because juice has no fiber and is high in sugar.

Milk group

Choose two servings per day from this group.

Toddler and preschooler
  1 cup milk
  1 cup yogurt
  2 slices processed cheese
  1 1/2 cups ice cream
  1 cup pudding
  1 1/2 sticks string cheese
  1 cup calcium-and-vitamin-D-fortified soy milk

Meat group

Choose two servings per day.

Toddler

1 1/2 ounces cooked lean meat
1 1/2 ounces chicken
1 1/2 ounces fish *or* 2 fish sticks
3/4 egg
3/4 hot dog* (cut in slices, not circles)
1 slice of luncheon meat
2 tablespoons of canned tuna
1/4 cup cooked beans
1/2 soy-burger patty

Preschooler

3 ounces cooked lean meat
3 ounces chicken or fish (*or* 4 fish sticks)
1 1/2 eggs
3 tablespoons peanut butter
1 1/2 hot dogs*
2 slices luncheon meat
1/3 cup canned tuna
3/4 cup beans
1/2 cup tofu
1 soy-burger patty

---

*I recommend nitrate-free, low-fat brands.

~

FYI: There are two easy ways to reduce fat in your preschooler's diet: (1) Gradually change from whole milk to low-fat milk by age five; and (2) offer lean meats or low-fat luncheon meats instead of hot dogs or bologna/salami. The entire family can follow these tips.

Sample Menu Ideas

The following are sample menus that reflect all nutritional requirements for toddlers and preschoolers. Do not expect your child to meet these goals every day. Be content if, on average over a week's time, your child gets most of it.

Toddler

Breakfast
> 1/2 slice toast
> 1/4 cup fruit juice
> 1/2 ounce cereal with 1/2 cup milk

Mid-morning snack
> 1 graham cracker
> 1/2 cup yogurt

Lunch
> 1 ounce meat
> 1/4 cup macaroni and cheese

2 slices cucumber

3 strawberries

1/2 cup water

Mid-afternoon snack

2 whole-grain crackers

1/2 tablespoon peanut butter

Dinner

1 1/2 ounces chicken

5 french fries

2 tablespoons ketchup

1/2 broccoli spear

1 bite of corn bread

1/2 cup milk

Preschooler

Breakfast

1/2 cup orange juice

1 slice whole-wheat toast with 1 teaspoon jam

1 ounce ready-to-eat fortified cereal with 1/2 cup low-fat milk and 1/4 cup blueberries

Mid-morning snack

1/2 bagel

1 stick string cheese

Lunch

1/2 cup applesauce

7 carrot sticks

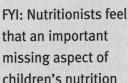

FYI: Nutritionists feel that an important missing aspect of children's nutrition could be remedied by adding a variety of vegetable and seed oils. Many essential fatty acids can be obtained by using small amounts of cooking oils, such as canola, safflower, sesame, and olive oils, to prepare food.

1/2 tuna-fish sandwich with a little mayonnaise
1/2 cup water

Mid-afternoon snack
1 cup air-popped popcorn
2 graham crackers
1 tablespoon peanut butter
1/2 cup low-fat milk

Dinner
1/2 cup spaghetti
3 small meatballs
1/2 cup sauce
1/2 cup of broccoli
1/2 cup ice cream

The Vegetarian Alternative

Vegetarian diets have been shown to significantly lower cholesterol levels and lead to lower adult risk of heart disease. Many of my patients have been reared without ever tasting meat. And they are doing just fine, thank you.

There is a Vegetarian Food Guide Pyramid created specifically for children (see illustration, page 133). The tip is the same as the one shown on the traditional pyramid. Fats and sweets are still advised in limited quantity. The big difference in this pyramid from the traditional food guide pyramid is the emphasis on vegetables, grains, and legumes. (Legumes are mostly beans: soy, pinto, kidney, peas, lima, lentils, garbanzo, and also soy proteins such as tofu.) The bottom level of the vegetarian pyramid suggests consuming at least one-third legumes and two-thirds whole grains in the diet. (Legumes represent about three servings and are a source of protein, healthful fat, and fiber.) Nuts and seeds are more important in a vegetarian diet, so your child needs about two servings from this category each day. Parents also need to choose cooking oils carefully. Oils are important, but they are left out of the standard pyramid because there is plenty of fat in meat and dairy. Choose vegetable oils.

Let me reassure you that your child can be reared as a vegetarian and be perfectly healthy. However, there are different kinds of vegetarians. The restrictive version that eliminates dairy products and eggs as well as animal protein from the diet (vegan) may represent special challenges for children under six years of age.

Certain nutrients *must* be supplied to your child's diet if you are rearing a little vegan. Vitamin B_{12} and iron are both essential to healthful growth and development. These nutrients can be provided in a vitamin/mineral supplement if you intend to avoid consuming milk and eggs. For these reasons, I recommend against vegan versions of vegetarianism for children and suggest including a variety of dairy products and eggs, even if mom and dad choose not to eat them. Feel free to discuss any concerns you have with your child's pediatrician.

Fortifying Foods: The Debate

It is increasingly common to find processed foods fortified with a variety of vitamins, minerals, and nutritional supplements. The argument is that we might as well fortify the foods children are most likely to eat, particularly breakfast foods. Many children will readily eat a Pop-Tart or a bowl of sweet breakfast cereal. When analyzed, it is often the fortified cereal at breakfast that provides the single largest contribution to a school-age child's daily nutritional needs. Some breakfast cereals are fortified with just about everything, for example, vitamins B, C, D, zinc, calcium, and folate. Our kids need all of those nutrients and more.

However, when cereal is fortified, choices have been made concerning what to fortify it with. Not only are unprocessed foods rich in folate and zinc, but these "real" foods also have myriad nutrients. In nature, food has small amounts of nutrients that we don't even know how to identify, much less duplicate. We are learning that many of these so-called *micronutrients* play vital roles in the prevention of disease and the maintenance of good health. Real food also offers nutrients in the forms that are ideal for absorption by the body.

Therefore, the argument against processed fortified foods asserts that, if we fill up our children with foods high in sugar appeal, we leave less room for other "whole," unprocessed foods. The problem with this argument is that most of the time our kids are eating low-nutrient, high-density, high-calorie foods anyway, not fresh fruits and vegetables, and the solution may be to fortify the foods that they *do* eat. Offer whole-grain, minimally processed foods in your child's diet to get him accustomed to eating these foods. If you are facing a temporary rebellion against such foods, then at least choose a fortified processed food.

11

The Good and Bad "Moos"
About Milk

The ABCs of Milk

Milk plays a prominent role in feeding infants, toddlers, and preschoolers. Milk is what we feed babies when they are born—it is the substance of life-giving nutrition. We use the phrase "mother's milk" not only to literally mean mother's milk but also figuratively to encompass all that is important to our well-being.

In the first six months of life, milk is almost all your child needs nutritionally. After that, milk should be only one part of your child's nutritious diet. We are the only mammals that continue to drink milk after weaning off breast milk. Babies need breast milk because it contains antibodies that provide protection from certain illnesses. It also offers carbohydrates, protein, and fats in a ratio that is vital for normal development of the human body. In particular, the fat in breast milk is beautifully designed by Mother Nature. It enhances the healthy development of the nervous system. These fats are called essential fats.

After weaning, milk requirements decrease rapidly. Although a typical infant needs about 32 ounces of milk a day, a typical two-year-old needs half that amount. Milk continues to be a good source of protein, a good source of "good" fat, and an easily available source of calcium and vitamin D. These nutrients can also be obtained by eating a combination of other foods. However, a child who overfeeds on milk usually has no "room" for these other foods.

> *Mrs. Smith and sixteen-month-old Justin just arrived for his checkup. She's excited about sharing Justin's accomplishments. After a routine complete blood count, I see that Justin is anemic, probably has iron-deficiency anemia. I ask, "What does Justin eat?" Mrs. Smith announces, "Well, I certainly make sure Justin gets enough milk every day."*
> *"How much is that?"*
> *"At least two quarts."*
> *"That's the likely source of his anemia."*

Although we all seem to know that "milk does a body good," many parents don't know that too much milk can actually do a body harm. As important as milk is (just look at all those popular "Got milk?" ads with celebrities and their milk mustaches), there are many misunderstandings about milk. The calcium in milk interferes with the body's absorption of iron. Additionally, milk can be difficult to digest, causing tiny losses of blood from the lining of the intestines. If sixteen-month-old Justin depends on milk for his nutrition to the exclusion of other foods, he may develop iron-deficiency anemia.

Myth: The More Milk, the Better

Children do not need to drink milk in huge quantities in order to receive enough calcium. A toddler typically needs no more than 16 ounces of milk to get all the calcium in a day that he needs. One ounce of cheese provides the same amount of calcium as 4 ounces of milk. If your child ate four slices of cheese a day, she would get all the calcium she needed without drinking a sip of milk.

Too much milk can be dangerous for your toddler. Let me state it again, because this may come as news to you: As wonderful as milk can be, too much milk irritates the gut and causes iron-deficiency anemia (and other nutrient deficiencies, such as copper.) Too much milk for a toddler is more than 16 ounces a day. (The only milk product that does not cause anemia is yogurt.) There are children who drink more than a quart (32 ounces) of milk a day. Children with iron-deficiency anemia often drink even more milk than that.

I see a lot of Mrs. Smiths. They come into my office and are proud to share with me how much milk their child drinks. They cannot understand how *their* child could possibly be anemic. When I explain how two quarts of milk a day can lead to anemia, parents commonly react first with shock and then embarrassment. There is no need to feel embarrassed; most

> The absorption of iron is enhanced by breast milk. However, breast milk is deficient in vitamin D and must be supplemented. (All infant formula and commercially available milk is fortified with vitamin D.)

people don't know that milk can have a "downside" that leads parents to create a problem unintentionally. The important thing is to fix the problem once a parent has been made aware of it.

Myth: Young Children Need Nonfat Milk So They Won't Get Fat

Mr. Brown brings in Allison for her eighteen-month checkup. I show dad how nicely Allison fits on the growth curve—the large end of the norm. Dad announces that he has been worried Allison might be getting fat because he has some relatives who are obese. In fact, his mother pointed out that Allison was headed in that direction. So eight months ago, dad took it upon himself to put Allison on a low-fat diet that most notably included only nonfat milk products.

Whether or not Allison was headed for obesity, she was possibly headed toward malnutrition and potential learning and fine-motor difficulties.

One reason infants need milk is because it contains special fats. Mother's milk has the perfect fats for baby and in just the right amounts. Infants need those fats for the very important job of growing a normal, healthy nervous system in the first two years of life.

After the age of two, the fat in milk becomes less necessary for lining the nervous system, and by the time the child is in preschool, he can even have nonfat (skim) milk. You can start to wean down to 2 percent milk after age two, 1 percent at age three and nonfat milk by age four or five, especially if there is concern about family cholesterol problems or obesity.

All dairy products that you give your child in the second year of life should be whole-milk, not low-fat products. You just have to spend your child's second year of life with two different kinds of milk in your refrigerator.

If whole milk is good for my daughter, should I be giving her butter instead of margarine?
No. Milk fat is altered in the process of becoming butter. Butterfat can even interfere with the body's use of the special milk fat for nervous-system development. Feeding a child butter only adds calories, not good nutrition. Please note that butter isn't even in the milk group on the Children's Food Guide Pyramid (see Chapter 10, page 132).

> *Exception to whole milk:* Children with a strong family history of early heart disease (before age forty) may be put on restrictive diets that include 2 percent milk. This is done with careful monitoring by the pediatrician or a specialist in family cholesterol problems.

Common Milk-Related Issues

Because parents think children need to drink a lot of milk, they come up with all sorts of ways to get the milk to go down.

Chocolate milk

I give my child chocolate milk because he doesn't really like plain milk. Isn't that OK?
From a milk standpoint, there's nothing wrong with that. The milk is just fine. Unfortunately commercial chocolate milk contains a lot of sugar, and that's not good for your child's teeth

or appetite. It's better to add a little bit of cocoa powder to plain milk, which is only a fraction of what the manufacturers actually put in the shelf versions of chocolate milk.

Often when parents ask me this question, I stop and ask, "How much chocolate milk does your child drink?" Most of the time I find out that the intake is huge, and the parent is really saying, "My child doesn't get as much milk as *I* think she should get," which is a much greater amount than what the child actually needs. This discovery often leads me to the conclusion that there is no need to offer the child chocolate milk at all. The typical diet of a toddler who "doesn't drink milk" usually includes milk on cereal in the morning, macaroni and cheese for lunch, and yogurt snacks. In other words, she gets plenty of milk without drinking all that chocolate milk.

Got calcium?

My child doesn't drink milk or eat other dairy products. My neighbor gives her child a calcium supplement. Can't I just do that?

Yes, your child does need calcium for bone growth in the first few years of life—upward of 500 milligrams a day. If your child has no obvious source of calcium, you can encourage him to eat an egg a day (an egg contains lots of calcium), as long as there is no family history of high cholesterol, and use calcium-fortified

FYI: Despite the touted high calcium content of some green vegetables, your child would actually have to eat several platefuls of kale, for example, to get enough calcium from this source.

juices in moderation. However calcium supplements are not a bad idea for a child on an anti-milk campaign. They come in liquid and chewable forms—your doctor will guide you.

Vitamin D and milk

Vitamin D is essential for bone growth and other important body functions. Deficiency results in a painful, deforming condition known as rickets. Vitamin D is easily made in your skin with exposure to the sun. But because of the increasing incidence of skin cancer, we are urged to stay out of the sun or wear sunscreen. Our children are at particular risk of developing rickets unless they are given vitamin D supplements. Fortified milk is the best source of this essential vitamin and 16 ounces provides twice the minimum daily requirement.

> FYI: Only fortified milk has vitamin D. Other dairy products, such as cheese and yogurt, do not provide vitamin D, although they are rich in calcium.

My child is "allergic" to milk

Milk sometimes gets a bad reputation because parents decide their child is allergic to it. What parents often mean is that their child shows an *intolerance* to large amounts of milk. That's not the same as an allergy to milk and can lead to unnecessary dietary restrictions that are hard to live with.

Lactose intolerance has to do with the sugar portion of milk. It is different from an allergy. Lactose is the sugar in milk. In order to digest it, your body makes an enzyme called lactase. Many children don't have enough of this enzyme, so milk gives them gas and a stomachache.

If your child is lactose intolerant, your pediatrician will give you several solutions. One option is to offer lactose-reduced milk. Many commercial versions exist on the dairy shelves that are designed to handle this specific problem. You can also buy lactase tablets or drops to give your child before she eats milk products. Another solution is to offer yogurt. Yogurt doesn't contain lactose, and it still offers the calcium your child needs.

The milk-allergic child

Some children truly *are* allergic to milk. That is, they are allergic to the *protein* portion of cow's milk. You would know because your infant would have blood in his stool. If you breast-feed and *you* drink a lot of cow's milk, your doctor may advise you to stop drinking cow's milk to prevent it from being passed to your baby through your milk. If you use a formula based on cow's milk, you would be advised to change formula. A milk-allergic child can get extremely sick, even to the point of losing consciousness, if given dairy products. The pediatrician will advise special precautions if your child has a milk allergy.

12

Junk Food

Junk Food Defined

Junk food is food that is high in any or all of the following: fat, sugar, salt. *Any* food that concentrates the vast majority of its calories in fat, sugar, or salt is junk food. Highly processed foods are often "junky" because they are loaded with all three. Some people's definition of junk food also includes any food that has on its label ingredients that are impossible to pronounce (such as chemical additives).

I want to add to that definition: Junk food is food that interferes with the quest for a well-balanced diet. It is food that is so imbalanced that it becomes virtually impossible to rebalance the total daily nutrition. For instance, one small bag of potato chips is equivalent to two days' worth of salt for a two-year-old. How do you plan to feed your child anything else after he's had his bag of chips? Anything becomes junk if it is all your child eats, and he eats a lot of it. Even Popeye's spinach can become junk food if eaten in very large quantities because it's so high in sodium and potassium.

Junk food is often dressed up in healthful-looking packages, so be a critical consumer when you buy. Those clever marketers want you to buy their product, so many food manufacturers advertise foods as health foods that are not necessarily healthful at all. Some chips are advertised as "lower in fat"—but that doesn't mean they aren't loaded with salt, and they still contain considerable fat (just less than the popular alternative). Another example is carob ice cream or carob candy bars. These bars, which are not made with high-fat chocolate, still contain a large amount of sugar. Lower-fat claims for yogurt and muffins are often conveniently silent on the fact that these foods may be packing lots of sugar, despite being lower in fat. That's not desirable, either!

Sugar: Often in All the Wrong Places

Everybody knows that breakfast is the most important meal of the day. Parents who want to make healthful breakfast choices for their young kids are now confronted by a variety of sugary cereals and breakfast bars. An industry has "popped up" that creates fast-food breakfast to cater to the hurried family. Today many of the most widely available breakfast choices are not healthful in the least. They are, in fact, junk food because they are very high in fat, sugar, and salt. You have to choose what to eat very carefully these days to avoid having a junk-food breakfast.

A popular choice would be a fruit Pop-Tart, with icing. (In the fruit tart's defense, you might observe, "Look, it has apples in it." Chances are there is actually very *little* real apple in it.) In fact, it is very high in fat and has no fiber unless you specifically buy a bar that is made with whole-wheat flour. Then your child probably won't eat it.

Maybe your child wants cereal instead. Look out! The old campfire dessert of chocolate bars, graham crackers, and marshmallows—s'mores—now has been dressed up as a popular breakfast cereal: tiny little s'mores floating in (another breakfast possibility) strawberry-flavored milk. Oreo cookies are also available these days thinly disguised as cereal. Your child washes it down with cup of Hawaiian Punch (yes, it happens). This is taking "sugar and spice" to the limits at breakfast time or any time. And this is just the *start* of your little one's day. Breakfast is a weak link in the diet for many people, not just little children, and adults should model better food choices also. For better breakfast ideas, see the examples in the Food Guide Pyramid in Chapter 10.

The Low-Down About the Sugar High

Sugar has been repeatedly accused of making children hyperactive. All the current research shows that sugar is not guilty as charged. Scientific studies use really huge amounts of sugar, yet in test after test, they find no discernable differences in behavior after the sugar challenge. And it doesn't matter who does the evaluating. They have done these studies with teachers and with parents making the observations. They have done the so-called double-blind tests. You name it, and they never produce the impact parents describe.

> Dear Dr. Paula,
>
> Our son is four and a half and has been having behavior problems in school. A teacher suggested I stop all sugar. I did and this morning he was a perfect angel. Then he went to his cousin's house and had some chocolate kisses. He came home a

"wild man." Can sugar have that much of an impact?

Jake's mom

Dear Jake's mom,

It's not the chocolate kisses that are turning your Dr. Jekyll into a mini Mr. Hyde, trust me. Any food energizes a child, and so does active play with his cousin.

I can see all of you shaking your heads and saying, "If you saw *my* child after he ate jelly beans, you would change your mind." Well, no, I wouldn't. So what could possibly explain the change in behavior parents see? One possible explanation is a matter of timing. After playing, children remain wired for a time. Kids are also often given sugar at transition times like after school—just when the child can let go, and he often does. You may be overlooking the fact that *anytime* you eat you get more energy. It doesn't matter *what* you eat. People confuse the energy associated with a meal with something specific *in* the meal.

All food leads to energy when it is consumed. That's one good reason why it's not a good idea to feed your child just before bedtime. You don't want your child to have an energy boost just when you're hoping for sleep.

Dear Dr. Paula,

After lunch I loaded up my girls and headed to the grocery store. Julie was in the basket of the cart and Beth in the seat. They got their cookie treats from the bakery, and then it was up and down the aisles. They did great until checkout. Beth began demanding to walk, and I let her down. I was trying to load the groceries on the conveyor belt, and off she went. I went after her and found her grabbing the M&M bags from the candy display. I told her she already had a cookie and would get no M&Ms. She fell on the floor shrieking as loud as she could.

Beth's mom

Dear Beth's mom,

I think grocery stores should have a sign that says, "Warning: Enter with a toddler at your own risk." I recall learning to shop by phone when my kids were that age. The temptations were too great, and my solutions were shortsighted. Many of us might reason that if given a cookie early, Beth would be satisfied throughout the journey. Not likely. I recall a children's book I read to my kids. I always laughed nervously when the story began, "If you give a mouse a cookie . . ." The message here is that "sugar begets more sugar." Sugar makes us feel good. It makes us want more, and if we're in a grocery store surrounded by temptation, one little cookie only triggers the desire for another cookie. Poor Beth didn't have a biological chance. Those M&Ms were speaking to her at a gut level. On top of that, any attempt to reason with a toddler is met with shocking failure. Sorry, mom. Leave her home when you can, and offer her a stick of celery the next time you dare enter the portals of nutritional doom. The junk food practically leers at you from the grocery store shelves, begging to be taken home.

Sugar and ADHD

ADHD, attention deficit (hyperactivity) disorder, which has been identified in children in ever-increasing numbers in the last

~

FYI: Sugar

All sugar is sugar. There's no such thing as good or bad sugar. (It doesn't come with little black and white cowboy hats.) It doesn't matter if it's brown sugar, fructose sugar, honey, molasses, "table" sugar—it's all nutritionally the same.

Sugar causes tooth decay. Sticky foods such as jellybeans are even worse than chocolate because the sugar remains on the teeth longer. But even sugar from fruit, if nestled in the teeth, can lead to cavities. (Raisins are really a problem in this way!) Offer water or brush your child's teeth after eating.

twenty years, has also been attributed to the high-sugar diet we feed our young children. Some researchers, with very little actual data, have created an entire industry that caters to that belief. The vast majority of scientific research indicates quite unequivocally that, in fact, sugar does *not* alter a child's behavior. (The exception is one small study specifically measuring the impact of huge amounts of sugar on the behavior of children previously diagnosed with severe ADHD. Even this study showed only very limited impact.)

Salt: Leave It off the Table

The body's *need* for salt is carefully controlled by delicately balanced processes involving the body's kidneys and cardiovascular systems. In contrast, a *taste* for salt is actually regulated by how much salt we eat. In other words, the more salt we eat, the more salt we *want*, because our taste buds become used to its taste.

Here's what is important: For about 6 percent of all children, high salt intake is not well managed by the body and causes high blood pressure—which can lead to adult heart disease. A little-known fact is that excessive salt intake also interferes with the body's use of calcium and its ability to build strong bones. Since the taste for salt is mostly an acquired one, it's best to keep the salt shaker off the table.

Fortunately, it's fairly simple to keep salt intake to a manageable level. Approximately 80 percent of a typical American child's dietary salt is found in fast foods, chips, and commercially made sauces and soups. These are all foods that can be eliminated or reduced without compromising good nutrition for our children. By banning the salt shaker, choosing carefully at the grocery store, and decreasing at least half the amount of salt we use in cooking, our children's daily salt intake can be safely moderated.

Can sugar give my child diabetes?

Recent research shows that infants who are fed very high sugar diets may have a higher chance of developing diabetes before the age of ten, especially if there is a strong family history of this disease.

Good Fat, Bad Fat

More feared than understood, dietary fats are essential for normal, healthy growth and development. In fact, infants under six months of age need fully one-half of their daily calories to come from fat. Nature's best, breast milk, is composed of precisely that amount of fat. That's the good news.

The bad news is that fat leads to obesity, heart disease, and all manner of bad adult health disorders when too much of it is found in the diet. Recent evidence even links high fat intake during childhood to adult cancer of the colon, breast, and uterus. Fat also begets more fat. It's true; the body's fat cells actually make an enzyme that attracts more fat.

There are, however, different kinds of fat. The infamous cholesterol-producing type has received much attention. We know that high blood-cholesterol levels predispose us to clogged arteries and adult heart disease. But cholesterol represents only a small fraction of the fats found in foods.

There *are* good fats. The fats found in vegetable oils, such as canola, olive, and corn oil, are particularly good for children's brain development. They contain essential fatty acids that are linked to proper nervous system growth and regulation. These vegetable oils may be even *more* beneficial for decreasing the risk of heart disease later on in life than the widely promoted "polyunsaturated" types, such as sunflower and safflower oils.

And then there are the bad fats. The fat found in butter, margarine, and shortening (lard), often found in baked goods, should be strictly avoided, particularly in the first year of life. These fats actually interfere with the body's ability to use the good fats for the developing nervous system. Interference during this crucial period of development is being linked to a wide variety of developmental disorders of childhood, including

Recommended Percentage of Fat in Daily Calorie Intake by Age

Under 6 months	50%
6 to 12 months	40%
1 to 2 years	35%
2 to 6 years	30%
Adult	less than 30%

attention deficits with or without hyperactivity (ADHD or ADD) and pervasive developmental disorder (PDD).

Keep your child's fat intake limited to the levels recommended for his or her age and choose mostly monounsaturated and polyunsaturated types, such as those found in vegetable oils. Consult your child's doctor if a family history for early coronary disease exists.

Read Labels!

Want to get scared? Don't rent *Blair Witch*, just go to your pantry and pull out some food. You'll have the equivalent of *Scream* right in your kitchen. Talk about not being able to judge a book by its cover! Many foods are disguised and "cleaned up" by marketing magicians to *appear* healthful. Rarely does food come with banners declaring, "I'm junk food."

On the bright side, I am very grateful that every food sold in this country has to list its ingredients. Ingredients are listed in order of quantity, starting with the ingredient that is presen the highest concentration. You can also count on the "Nutrition Facts" label that must also appear by law on each commercial food product. If the ingredient list is in such tiny print you can't read it, that may be a warning in and of itself. Ask yourself: Do the manufacturers feel they have something to hide? Get out your magnifying glass and read anyway.

These foods came right out of my neighbor's pantry. (Don't tell her children's pediatrician!)

Strawberry fruit leathers.   This product shows marketing at its best, or worst, depending upon your view. The package I looked at declares, "This snack is made with real fruit, and is an excellent source of vitamin C." So far, it sounds fairly nutritious. So let's look at the ingredients. The first ingredient is "pears from concentrate." Wait a minute, this is a *strawberry* fruit leather! What if your child is allergic to pears? I can't pronounce the rest of the ingredients. It seems to me that a lot of thought went into the misleading packaging of this product.

Flavored corn tortilla chips.   These are slightly better than most chips, because the first ingredients are actually food: corn, vegetable oil, followed by corn oil, soybean oil, sunflower oil, buttermilk; then salt, tomato powder (there's the vegetable). And now comes a list of ingredients I can't pronounce, including MSG, malic acid, then various kinds of salts, and a gel—yellow dye #5, tartrazine, which is bad for your kid, especially if he is asthmatic—red dye, and still more ingredients. (I would have chosen those neon-colored puffs to examine, but that orange powder gets all over my clothes.)

ut butter.   Let's look at one major peanut butter acturer's label for creamy peanut butter with "fresh roasted peanuts." First of all, calling something "fresh" is just a marketing device. (Could you have a product with "rotten" roasted peanuts?) Peanut butter could be a healthful, high-nutrient, plant-protein food. Let's check the label on this jar: roasted peanuts and sugar (an unnecessary ingredient), partially hydrogenated vegetable oil, more and more oils, and so on.

There is really nothing necessary for making wonderful peanut butter except peanuts. Don't give up attempts to get kids to eat more healthfully. Take real peanut butter and mix it into your child's favorite brand. Gradually decrease the offending peanut butter and increase the pure-peanut peanut butter until you are using only the pure-peanut product.

Canned spaghetti and meatballs. This product is designed to be eaten by children. The can I looked at says that it is a "good source of body-building protein" and "contains no preservatives." Both of those claims turn out not to be true. The first ingredient is tomato sauce, then pasta. We don't get to the meat in the meatballs until *far* down the list, so clearly this isn't a good source of protein for your child.

At first glance, you might think your dairy-allergic child could eat this, but this product also contains "whey," pasteurized milk culture, and some cheddar cheese . . . probably not ingredients you would add if you made spaghetti and meatballs yourself. If you had bought this product, you probably would have thought your child was safe from ingesting dairy products, because this product declares itself "spaghetti and meatballs in tomato sauce," without mentioning the presence of cheese at all.

Canned foods like this one can present other problems. According to the label I looked at, the total fat in one cup of th spaghetti and meatballs was 11 grams per serving, and one serving is equal to only half of the can. Trust me, if your ch likes this stuff he will eat the entire can—for a whopping 22 grams of fat. Read further, and see that 90 calories per serving come from fat. The entire can represents 500 calories. What's more, the cholesterol in this can is 25 milligrams. The sodium content is 1,050 milligrams, which is far more than your child's entire daily allowance for this mineral. Ouch! (This "perfect and nutritious food," according to the manufacturer, meets *my* definition of junk food.)

Canned corned beef hash.   The corned beef hash I looked at came in an individual serving can (7.5 ounces). The label makes you think this product gives you one big protein boost. Corned beef hash does contain protein, but it also has more salt than any child should have (1,270 milligrams), as well as 65 milligrams of cholesterol, which is a lot. This tiny can contains a whopping 440 calories, with 290 of those calories contributed by fat. This represents almost one-half of your child's total daily caloric requirements, and it's mostly fat. With products like these, is it any wonder that 50 percent of our children are considered obese?

Lunch meat, cracker, and cheese packs with drink.   Often clearly marketed for children, this type of product may be fun to eat, but it's sure not very healthful. The drink component I looked at contains no more than 10 percent fruit juice. Although it calls itself "wild cherry," its label reveals that water, corn syrup, and pear juice from concentrate are the main ingredients. (There's pear again, filling in for other flavors!) The lunch I examined contained several crackers, bologna, a chunk of "cheese food," and a candy dessert. The calories on the package are listed as 530, with 240 of them contributed by fat. Further investigation of the ingredients list reveals that this lunch is loaded with saturated fat, cholesterol, 1,210 milligrams of salt, and 44 grams of sugar. Your children might indeed be willing, even eager, to eat this if you were to pack it into their lunch boxes, but it gets my junk food seal of disapproval.

I suggest as an alternative to your usual rainy day activities taking the time to pull out foods already on your pantry shelves and read the labels. Be ready to go shopping afterward!

It's Not All Junk!

There's good news too. Some foods you may characterize as junk may not be. Let's take a look at some surprisingly nutritious quick foods.

Popcorn.   Popcorn often gets lumped in with chips, but it offers far fewer calories from fat. Popcorn, in fact, is *not* junk food unless it's drowned in butter or salt. If your kids are already hooked on popcorn, teach them to use less butter by mixing your child's preferred brand with a little more air-popped popcorn each day.

Pizza.   Parents often think that pizza is junk food, maybe because kids like it so much. Pizza is often convenient and can be healthful. It's a serving of cheese, a serving of tomato sauce and a serving of bread. A slice of pizza, maybe even two, is not junk food. Consider some veggie toppings and blot off the grease with a paper towel before serving. Also, you're on your honor here: Obviously a pizza that is loaded with sausage, or that comes with a crust that is stuffed with additional chees not a smart nutritional choice for your child or anybody else. Keep pizza simple!

Grilled fast foods.   Your child can eat a relatively healthful meal even at a fast food place like McDonald's. The grilled chicken sandwich is fine. So is the turkey Caesar salad cup. Even McDonald's is trying to hop on the healthier-food bandwagon—some restaurants offer the new McVeggie Burger. Let me tell you what's *not* a healthful meal at McDonald's: french fries with a standard double cheeseburger and a McFlurry shake. With the fat, sugar, and salt in all of that, your child is in big nutritional trouble.

Avoid the fat toppings.   You can always ruin a good thing. The ads tout the goodness of a Subway-brand sandwich, but if you let them add the standard dousing of olive oil, salt, and mayonnaise or butter on the roll, then you have lapsed into the junk food category.

Ketchup.   A lot of kids will eat healthful food if it's covered in ketchup. However, a lot of parents think ketchup is junk food. In excess, it can be. But if you have to choose among ketchup, mayonnaise, or your child not eating at all, allow the ketchup.

Ice cream.   Sometimes ice cream is junk food, and sometimes it isn't. Specialty brands are extremely high in fat, and yes, it must be admitted, in flavor. Ice creams that have natural flavors are often on the lower end of butterfat percentages and can be healthful in moderation. Check out the old-fashioned flavors of regular Breyer's (not the specialty "gourmet" line), which prides on all-natural ingredients that you can even pronounce.

Keep in mind that no matter how careful you are about banning junk food and serving healthful meals, "junky" foods *do* creep in—maybe from grandmother's house or in the form of a birthday goodie bag. An occasional fall off the "cookie wagon" won't hurt!

13

The Couch Potato
and Childhood Obesity

We're raising a generation of little spuds who are on the road to becoming full-grown adult potatoes. The couch potato is the child who sits on the couch—or chair, or floor—watching TV with his finger glued to the remote control. Some kids' only regular exercise is channel surfing. (We don't even get up any more to turn channels on the TV.) The average American child, age six to ten, watches six hours of television a day. (Ouch!) Children are becoming conditioned to inactivity at the same time they are "feasting" on all those ads for junk food. It's a terrible combination.

We are a nation of sedentary people destined to get even more sedentary. We are looking at a future of moving sidewalks, a future in which education won't even require attending school—the child can "go to school" on his home television/computer system. With the entertainments available today, including computer games, time spent on-line, television shows, videos, and DVDs, we are guaranteeing future generations of sedentary obese people.

Actually, the future is now. Childhood obesity is epidemic—and it's a proven precursor to adult obesity. Adults who are obese are more likely to suffer from high blood pressure, heart attacks, stroke, arthritis, diabetes, broken bones, and more. All of these conditions are induced or worsened by obesity. Some obesity is related to genetics, but most of it is directly related to lifestyle and nutrition.

Obesity Defined

Overweight is a term defined as increased body size. *Obesity*, however, is defined as having excess body fat. Not every overweight person is obese. Health professionals are very concerned about obesity because it is linked to a variety of debilitating adult diseases, such as high blood pressure and diabetes.

Obesity is often judged subjectively by a person's appearance. But there are objective measures that strictly define this condition. Special growth charts, which are found in every pediatrician's office, compare children's heights to their weights. If your child is 20 percent heavier than the average child of the same height, he is considered obese. In 1994, almost 50 percent of American children were found to be obese by this criterion in a national survey.

The Link Between Television and Obesity

Did you know that the more television one watches and the more computer and video games one plays, the more likely one to be obese? In 1998, 65 percent of Americans "qualified" for definition of obesity. Watching television or videos may lly appear harmless, but it affects behavior. A parent will say to me, "But my daughter dances to *Barney* and her eyes just sparkle." Studies of infants placed in front of television programs tell a different story. These studies show the babies paying little or no attention to the television at first. After only six weeks of exposure, they decrease their physical activity by a whopping *80 percent*. So the same baby who started off dancing to *Sesame Street* and singing along with *Teletubbies* is now sitting motionless, staring at the screen.

You see the same phenomenon among adults *in* restaurants and sports bars that have television screens. People's conversations slow down. The person facing the television is a goner, while the less fortunately seated dinner date will soon find themselves talking to the wall. When people watch television, there is a measurable change in their brain-wave activity—it slows. Whenever we let that happen, we have taken the first steps toward losing the battle of the bulge.

When Should I Worry About My Child's Weight?

Dear Dr. Paula,

Jonah is eating us out of house and home (not really)! He is eight months old and eats as much as I do. I swear he would never stop if I didn't just "close the kitchen" after the third jar. Is he going to end up really fat? No one in my family is fat.

Jonah's mom

Dear Jonah's mom,

You have a "barracuda" on your hands. Chances are he will grow up healthy and hearty. Don't try to curb his naturally large appetite, but be particularly careful to avoid junk foods, and encourage him to be an

active child. Skip the "boob tube" and head for the
playground. Don't overreact and never try to put him
on a diet.

The role of temperament

Some children are born with temperaments that may put them
at higher risk for obesity. The infant who always sucks the
bottle dry, what I call "the barracuda," or the older baby who
starts solid foods and stuffs everything into her mouth ("the
stuffer") may require you to pay a little more attention to the
foods you offer.

Infants are supposed to be chubby

Your well-fed, chubby-looking four-month-old is no more likely
to be a fat adult than is her sleek-looking counterpart. Children
in the first year of life, if they are fed a healthful diet, are not
classified as obese with rare exceptions. Babies less than one
year old often have that "Pillsbury doughboy" look. It's cute!
(Don't forget: *Infants don't belong on diets.*) A normal infant
needs to eat approximately 100 calories per kilogram a day. (A
20-pound baby needs about 900 calories a day, and a 10-pound
baby needs no more than 450 daily calories.) So even if your
baby is in the 90th percentile and has more folds than a shar-pei
puppy, your child is *not* obese.

Activity Defeats Obesity

~~ivity~~ and childhood go together like hugs and kisses, which is
~~~, a lot of activity is good for your little one. Exercise
~~~s important once a child is able to walk and move. The

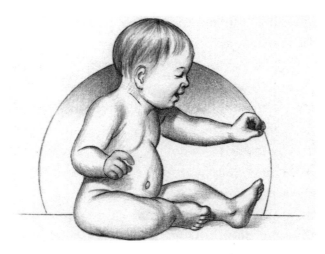

one-year-old who is parked in front of the television instead of roaming around after Mom is on his way to obesity. A fat two-year-old (whose growth chart position is greater than the 95th percentile) is likely to be a fat adult.

Your child needs the freedom and the opportunity to move about. Exercise is not only for keeping the balance between the calories eaten and the calories burned for energy and growth, it also stimulates your body to produce hormones for digestion and for production of endorphins, the "feel-good" hormones. Movement can also produce self-confidence. ("Wow, I caught that ball!") Muscles develop *only* in response to use. If you don't use them, you are abusing them. You can't easily make up for this missed opportunity later on.

Rules to Live By

1. Avoid parking your kids in front of the television (also known as the electronic baby-sitter).

2. If you missed Rule 1: Never feed your child in front of the television. The ads on television are geared to sending your

messages that say, "Buy me and eat me"—and your child is likely to become an overeater.

3. Turn off the television and the computer. Beware of all electronic devices claiming to be educational. Some of them may teach your child math. Your child will have ample opportunities to learn math once he goes to school. The price you pay for teaching him math early is a dulling of the brain and a slowing of reflexes; the only thing that truly expands as a result is your child's body, not his mind.

4. Go out and play! Your child will learn more about life by interacting with it directly. Going to the park teaches a child to compromise with the other children he meets, to stand up for himself, and to share. These are valuable life lessons he can't get from television. Your child's activity level outdoors may surprise you if you're used to a docile child sitting in front of a television. He will not sit still outside unless you put a Game Boy in his hand, in which case that device will act like an adhesive that glues him to the seat. Get your child a soccer ball instead, and turn him or her into a *real* Game Boy or Girl, not a virtual one.

> FYI: Girls are at a greater risk of inactivity than boys, so be careful not to direct your daughter away from the playground.

5. Don't be a parent who encourages your child to be an observer. You can create a couch potato by sitting in the park with your child in the stroller. Some children by their nature will be observers rather than participants, but don't encourage it. Look for activities your child is more likely to join, and when necessary, give a little push in the right direction.

6. Modeling is vital. Your child is not likely to give up being a couch potato unless *you* go first. Find activities you can share with your child. The younger they are, the easier that is, because they will do almost anything you do. If you feel like going swimming, take your baby with you. (Be aware that if you are jogging with your infant in the stroller, however, only you are getting exercise.)

My Child Is Fat. Now What?

Dear Dr. Paula,

Help! We have a real sumo wrestler. Barry is four years old, weighs 65 pounds, and hardly moves. My wife's family are all "big-boned" people, and they think Barry is just fine. I think they're dreaming and Barry is obese. What do you think?

Sumo wrestler's dad

Dear Sumo wrestler's dad,

You are probably right about Barry heading for trouble. The tendency toward obesity can run in families. Start now by turning off the television and video games and head outdoors—every day. Also consult with a pediatric nutritionist soon, and have your child's cholesterol checked. Your pediatrician can guide you, but don't wait. Finally, please be sensitive to your son's feelings; you should avoid cute labels like "sumo wrestler" anywhere within his earshot. Emotions play a large part in some children's food behavior.

Once a child is identified as obese, a parent's job is to work with a pediatrician and maybe enlist assistance from a pedia

~

Obesity Facts: A Summary

- Three in five children are now overweight.
- Our children consume too many of their daily calories from fat.
- Children are avid television watchers.
- Television watching is a prelude to obesity.
- Childhood obesity continues into adulthood.

nutritionist. Some suggestions are obvious; for instance, if your child is sitting in front of the television, you need to change that behavior and provide opportunities for fun exercise. Here are some suggestions for children under age six:

- Don't rush to put your child on a diet. At young ages, diets just don't work. They lead to lowered self-confidence and sneaky food behaviors.
- Increase physical activity rather than decrease food intake.
- See what your child is really eating. Keep a food diary.
- Model good eating habits.
- Never blame the child for his or her weight.
- Never talk about a weight problem in front of your child.
- Encourage physical activity by modeling.

14

Is Our Food Safe? Pesticides, Preservatives, Additives, and Germs

The food we eat is mostly *very* safe. Scientists have concluded that the risks of the foods we eat with regard to pesticides, hormones, and additives are small when compared to the risks of food spoilage and bacterial contamination. Unfortunately, dangerous bacterial contamination is not that uncommon. Fortunately, there is something *you* can do about the latter, and the government does a lot about the former.

People want to know: Are pesticides, preservatives, or additives like food coloring bad for you? The not-so-simple answer is, They could be, but the government maintains incredibly strict regulations for approval for any new food color, pesticide, or additive. In fact, foods that are in the "all natural" category and have no pesticides or additives are sometimes the source of serious bacterial infections and even fatalities. For example, raw natural honey sometimes turns out to be not so sweet. It may contain *botulinum* spores, which can cause a fat

∽

Raw natural honey sometimes turns out to be not so sweet. It may contain botulinum *spores, which can cause a fatal infection in infants. This is the reason we pediatricians don't let you put honey into baby's formula.*

infection in infants. This is the reason we pediatricians don't let you put honey into baby's formula.

Rigid testing goes into establishing safe exposure levels to additives, preservatives, and pesticides. It takes ten years to complete the process of getting permission to use a new pesticide or additive in our food. Translation: A mere *one* in 20,000 new pesticide products actually makes it from the lab to the farmer's field and ultimately to your salad bowl.

I take the view that the government is mostly very good about protecting our food, and although there is potential for problems with anything you add to food, most additives are carefully evaluated. *The bottom line is that we have the safest food in the world.*

∽

We have the safest food in the world.

There are circumstances when food available in U.S. markets may contain unsafe levels of toxic chemicals. Americans consume considerable amounts of imported produce, some of which has been found to contain unacceptable levels of prohibited or strictly controlled substances. Although the USDA attempts to check all imported foods carefully, some may slip by. I would suggest that, as a parent of young children, you read labels carefully and, unless unavoidable, only "buy American."

Pesticides

Pesticides are meant to control pests and plant diseases that threaten crops and food supplies. Parents are understandably concerned about pesticides appearing in the foods their children eat. The prevailing logic is, "I won't give my kid a food that's sprayed with something that's meant to kill bugs. If it can kill bugs, it can kill my kid." Wrong. There are strict regulations involved in testing pesticides for their safety in humans, overseen by the Food and Drug Administration (FDA), which works closely with the Environmental Protection Agency (EPA). The professionals in these government agencies are not trying to poison us.

On the other hand, infants and children may be especially sensitive to potential health risks posed by pesticides. In large quantities (not the quantities you can ingest by eating sprayed

Real Food Dangers

Beware: In the effort to look for additive-free, preservative-free, or pesticide-free food, you may fall into the trap of not realizing *true* dangers that lurk in food. There are toxins out there. *E. coli,* for example, can show up in anything uncooked, such as red meat; *salmonella* can show up in mayonnaise—it comes uninvited to picnics—and hepatitis is associated with seafood contamination.

foods), pesticides may cause damage to the central nervous system and have been implicated in some forms of cancer and respiratory illness. The EPA, responding to the 1993 National Research Council Review of potential risks to children due to pesticides, has undertaken extensive studies known as STAR (Science to Achieve Results) to assess any special vulnerability of children to pesticides.

Young children are potentially more vulnerable to pesticides for several reasons:

- Their internal organs are still maturing, and exposure to a toxin may permanently alter the way a child's biological system operates.
- Children's organs may absorb chemicals more readily than those of adults and be less able to break them down and excrete them from their bodies.
- In relation to their body weight, infants and children eat and drink more than adults, possibly increasing their exposure to pesticides in food and water.
- Pesticides may block the absorption of important food nutrients essential for normal, healthy growth.
- Certain behaviors, such as crawling on floors, playing outdoors, and putting objects in their mouths, increase children's exposure to pesticides.

A 1995 EPA report, "Pesticides in the Diets of Infants and Children," summarizes the need for more research, despite the encouraging findings that "no specific harm to children could be attributed to any pesticide when appropriately used." Areas of concern remain, particularly in regard to children who grow up and around agricultural communities, where pesticide exposure may be increased, and to the potential for accidental ingestion.

There are several things you can do to minimize the risk of pesticide exposure:

- Wash and scrub fruits and vegetables to remove pesticide residue. Unfortunately not all pesticides can be removed by washing.
- Peel fruits and vegetables, as pesticides rarely infiltrate beneath the skin.
- Trim fat from meat, and remove the skin of poultry and fish. Pesticides may collect in these places.
- Select a variety of foods to avoid repeated exposure to the same pesticide.

Food Additives

Food additives are defined as *any* substance added to food. "Additives" are an umbrella label including everything from sugar and salt to food colorings to aspartame. Even common ingredients that are added to keep food fresh, prevent spoilage, and add flavor are considered additives.

Food additives are also regulated by the government. Only minimal quantities are allowed in foods, and the additives have to be listed on the food label. Every proposed additive goes through rigid review procedures, which sift out the potential bad guys. For example, the Food and Safety Inspection Service outlawed the use of sorbic acid because it can make food *appear* to be fresh, even if spoilage has occurred. Although sorbic acid itself is safe, it can mask an unsafe situation, and for that reason the licensing bureau refused to approve it for use as an additive

Why do we use additives? The most common reasons are to preserve food quality, improve nutritional values, keep foods fresh, and slow microbial growth in food, preventing spoilage.

If we go through the common additive list, maybe we can "subtract" some of the concern you may feel about additives. Today some additives are under a literal, as well as figurative, microscope for possible unhealthful side effects.

BST (bovine somatotropin) is a hormone added to the diet of cows to increase milk production. Some parents are opposed to its use for fear that it could affect the children who drink induced milk. BST is a bovine hormone, and there is no scientific evidence that consuming BST-stimulated-cow milk affects children's hormone levels or development in any way.

Nitrates and nitrites are combinations of nitrogen and oxygen, which are naturally occurring chemicals found in soil. They are also natural components of the foods we eat. They help preserve color and prevent spoilage in food. There is no proof that these chemicals are bad for us. The bottom line is that consuming nitrates and nitrites is unavoidable, because these substances are even found in organic foods. Nitrates and nitrites have been accused of causing cancer, but no scientific jury has ever convicted them for this. However, if repeatedly brought to very high temperatures (as in frying bacon), some nitrites become compounds called nitrosamines and nitrosamides. In large quantities, these compounds have been found to be carcinogens. Rendered animal fat from processed meats can be high in these substances (see box on facing page).

Sulfites are an additive that helps food maintain a fresh appearance. Asthmatics may be sensitive to sulfites and should avoid them. It can be anywhere in foods, but mostly it is found light-colored fruits and vegetables to prevent darkening. Read ls.

~

About Rendered Fat

Bacon is not a particularly healthful food. It may taste good, but it is high in fat, salt, and nitrates. If you crave bacon, then fry up a slice or two (if you must), but don't save the bacon grease so you can cook french fries in it later. "Rendered" fat is particularly likely to contain carcinogenic nitrosamines.

Monosodium glutamate is an additive that is used as a flavor enhancer. It is deemed safe for adults, but we don't know if it's safe for kids. MSG is linked to "Chinese food syndrome," since it is often added to Chinese foods. It can cause headaches, a flushed face, and sudden disorientation. If you go to a Chinese restaurant, just say, "No MSG in my food, please."

Once there were dozens of *food dyes;* now there are just a handful. Tartrazine, yellow food dye, is one of the very few food dyes left. Some kids are allergic to it and may break out in hives and suffer from itching. People allergic to aspirin are most often affected. If you notice a connection between yellow food, such as yellow Jell-O or orange soda, and your child breaking out in an itchy rash, it could well be that tartrazine is the culprit. Tartrazine must be listed on the ingredients list on the label, so you can simply read labels in the grocery store and avoid bringing it home.

Aspartame is added as a sweetener to many foods children eat. Aspartame appears to increase seizures in children with petit mal epilepsy (also known as absence seizures). In additio children report increased occurrence of headaches after drinking aspartame-sweetened drinks.

Additives and hyperactivity

One controversy surrounding additives is what part, if any, they play in causing *hyperactivity*. Few medical problems have generated such emotion on the part of parents and teachers as hyperactivity, which is estimated to affect 3 to 15 percent of all U.S. children. A variety of ingredients, such as additives, food colorings, preservatives, and even certain trace minerals, have all been reported in the lay press and occasionally in the scientific literature to be linked to the development of ADHD. Scientists have concluded that there is no proof that giving children food with additives affects their activity level.

Sensible Food Practices: Fighting Germs

Although food that spends a few seconds on a clean floor or that is passed between two healthy children is unlikely to cause any harm if it is eaten, some very serious illnesses are caused by contaminated food. What follows are practical tips for keeping your food safe.

FYI: If you need another reason to avoid hot dogs, know that a certain dangerous bacteria known as *listeria* is commonly found in these processed meats. *Listeria* is otherwise mostly found only in animal feces.

Wash and scrub all fresh fruits and vegetables, particularly those that will be eaten uncooked. A simple diluted solution of vinegar and water is effective and inexpensive. This will help remove bacteria and traces of many chemicals.

Be a picky shopper. Some food choices have fewer additives than others, so read labels carefully.

Limit the use of packaged or processed convenience foods. Remember, you'll find more high-calorie, low-nutrient-density food in packaged and processed food than you will find in food you put together yourself. Why? Because we don't routinely add starch or sugar when we're cooking. And if we do, it's just a pinch. Choose fresh meat and poultry products instead of cold cuts and processed meats, which are high in various additives.

Choose foods that look healthful. For instance, when you buy corn, peel back the husk to look at it; it should appear shiny and moist, and the hairs inside should still be yellow. If they're black, that's mold—don't bring it home. If any food looks unhealthful, never taste it to find out. Some toxins are so poisonous that even a small taste can cause serious harm. Trust your instincts and toss the food.

Always wash your hands before you handle food. The less you handle food the better. Use sealed-tight containers to store leftovers and then refrigerate.

Keep hot foods hot and cold foods cold. Avoid letting cooked food cool down or warm up except by refrigeration or direct heat. Food allowed to sit at temperatures between 40° and 140°F may become contaminated and harmful to your health, particularly to your children's health, as their smaller size makes any germ ingestion potentially more dangerous. Discard any food that has spent over an hour outdoors or two hours in a cool environment.

Thaw frozen food in the refrigerator, not on the counter. If you're thinking about defrosting food from the freezer, store the food in small portions so that you don't have to refreeze unused portions after it's been defrosted. Refreezing can lead to bacterial contamination. When putting meats in the freezer, label them with the date.

Organize your kitchen cabinet so that newer foods are in the back. Put fresh foods, which usually last three days, up front.

Cook meat thoroughly; do not eat pink meat. Insert the meat thermometer in several places in the meat you cook before you decide it's at the right temperature for doneness. Portions of the meat may have cold spots that are undercooked. Bacteria reside in undercooked meat.

Store canned foods safely. Canned foods generally remain safe unless they're exposed to heat above 100°F (78°C). Some cupboards reach 100°F during the summer. If that is a possibility in your area, put a thermometer on the shelf in the pantry and periodically check the temperature. Reconsider the storage of your canned goods in the summer, when it can get really hot, or take the doors off the cabinet so that air will circulate around the cans. Look for signs of spoilage, such as cans that are leaking or bulging. Throw them away!

Always vigorously wash your work surfaces with warm, soapy water after use, especially cutting boards, because food residue gets into cracks and germs can grow there. Use separate boards for cutting raw meat.

Avoid eating undercooked or raw meat or eggs. When baking, do not allow your child to lick the bowl if raw eggs have been added to the batter.

Young children should avoid eating raw fish, even fish that is meant to be eaten raw, as in sushi. Children can get hepatitis from just a small amount of infected raw fish.

Never feed your baby directly from the baby-food jar if you're thinking of keeping leftovers for later. If the spoon went back in the food after it went in the baby's mouth, throw out the leftover food; it's contaminated. Don't let your children "double dip." If they put their finger into the peanut butter jar and lick it off, they must not repeat the performance, or you must dump the rest.

Let's face it, you can't spray away *all* the pests in your children's lives. There is no need to be the health food police, on twenty-four-hour alert. Just follow my guidelines and your own good common sense.

The Last Word . . .

Just like the creature under the bed and the ghost in the closet, your little dessert monster and fast-food fanatic is likely to disappear over the years.

In keeping with my beliefs, I prescribe, as always, a large dose of patience and a big spoonful of humor (not sugar, for obvious reasons). Even with the best planning and recipes, sometimes all your child will eat is an all-day sucker, two crayons, and some fruit punch. And even occasional breaches of the "Ten Food Commandments" are unlikely to lead to permanent nutritional disaster. As parents, we should be concerned with all aspects of our children's health and never lose sight of life's most important goal: rearing happy, healthy children. Bon appétit!

Acknowledgments

Thank you to my wonderful children David (cabbage eater!) and Shira (Cookie Dough monster that you are!), even though only one of you slept easily through the nights! You are always my best inspirations.

Thanks to all the wonderful parents I have been fortunate to work with and to all your creative children and to the endless uneaten meals we tried. Special thanks to the wonderful moms on the Web site www.drpaula.com (especially IS—G-d bless you and yours!) and the kitchen sink crowd for sharing your stories, your glories and your defeats.

Thank you Nancy Fish—for the smiles, for the hugs, for the enduring support.

Last and certainly not least: The task of writing this book could not even have been imaginable were it not for the sisterhood and loving friendship I am privileged to share with Linda Lee Small. You are in every line of this work (yes, literally), and you are in every fond thought of my mind. You are truly the master of the two-minute meal. I love you very much. See you at the spa.

Index